# Social Innovations in Urban Sanitation in India

This book discusses effective social innovation strategies facilitated by civil society organisations (CSOs) to tackle India's significant urban sanitation challenge. It presents the contours of an ecosystem that includes citizen participation and strengthening community-managed systems for improved sanitation and public health.

The book analyses case studies of effective sanitation programmes as well as experiments with innovative ideas in different regional contexts by CSOs to meet the contextual needs of the community and to ensure access to safe sanitation, especially among the urban poor. It highlights the challenges and the need for active participation of communities for change in behaviour, increasing institutional capacities of municipalities and standardising and scaling up strategies which work. The authors highlight the need for designing low-cost solutions, organising informal sanitation workers, serving marginalised communities and building effective alliances between communities and institutions to influence public policy.

Rich in empirical data, this book will be useful for officials of cities, public policymakers, scholars and researchers of urban studies, public policy, governance, political science, development studies and sociology as well as for CSOs and non-governmental organisations (NGOs) working on urban sanitation, urban planning and public policy.

**Shubhagato Dasgupta** is a Senior Fellow at the Centre for Policy Research (CPR) and Director of the Scaling City Institutions for India (SCI-FI) programme. His research focuses on low-income housing, drinking water and sanitation in India and the world, with particular reference to flagship government programmes and service delivery challenges in smaller cities. In the past he has worked in research and the practice of urban development in institutions including Housing and Urban Development Company, Infrastructure Development Finance Company, the World Bank and the International Finance Corporation. He has more than 40 publications on topics of water, sanitation, urban infrastructure and service delivery financing, housing and slum rehabilitation, urban sector public finance, and urban environmental infrastructure planning, management, and investment alternatives.

**Kaustuv Kanti Bandyopadhyay** is the Director of Participatory Research in Asia (PRIA) and Head of PRIA International Academy (PIA). He has 30 years of experience with the university, research institutions and civil society. He has led numerous participatory research and action learning initiatives to strengthen citizen participation in democratic governance using participatory planning, monitoring, evaluation and social accountability in urban and rural contexts. He is an acclaimed researcher and adult educator with expertise in organisation development, participatory monitoring and evaluation, participatory training methodologies and participatory research. He has extensively worked in India and other Asian countries. He has authored several articles, manuals, books and publications, which contributed to knowledge on participatory governance and strengthening civil society in Asia. He has a PhD in Anthropology for his work with the Parhaiya tribes of Chotanagpur in India.

**Anju Dwivedi** is an Associate Fellow at the Centre for Policy Research (CPR) working with the Project on Scaling City Institutions for India (SCI-FI): Sanitation. Her work includes supporting communities and state and urban local bodies with inclusive approaches to sanitation. She has carried out ethnographic research on culture and sanitation in small towns which has been published in the journal. She has done research on capacity-building needs of ULBs in small towns on sanitation and gender and urban sanitation. She has a master's in Social Anthropology, and before joining CPR, she worked with the Support to National Policies for Urban Poverty Reduction Project, a partnership between DFID and the Ministry of Housing and Urban Poverty Alleviation to support the development of pro-poor urban policies (housing and livelihood in 20 cities across 15 states). She has 28 years of experience in the development sector, in both rural and urban areas, and worked with communities, local governance institutions and civil society groups.

**Sumona DasGupta** is a political scientist by training with a special interest in South Asian politics, governance, democracy and dialogue, peace and conflict. She is a Research Advisor to Women in Security Conflict Management and Peace, a member of the Calcutta Research Group (CRG), an association of scholar-activists working on democracy, human rights peace and justice, and serves on the board of editors of the *International Feminist Journal of Politics* and is guest editor of *Peace Prints*, a South Asian journal of peacebuilding. She is a published author with Routledge, among others, who has written extensively on issues related to dialogue, deepening democracy and conflict resolution. Her book *Citizen Initiatives and Democratic Engagements: Experiences from India* was published by Routledge in 2010.

**Bharti** is a Development Professional and worked as a Senior Research Associate at the Centre for Policy Research (CPR). Her Research focused on the issues of equity and inclusion, governance, capacity building and community participation across both urban and rural water and sanitation space. In the past, she has worked on projects of water governance, water management, water policies, housing for the poor, low-cost housing microfinance, cooperatives and rural livelihoods with institutions like the World Bank, the Food and Agriculture Organisation (FAO), UN, Deloitte, central, state and local governments, think tanks, research institutes and community-based organisations. Her area of work primarily concerns policy review, qualitative and quantitative research, project management, economic and financial analysis, business sustainability, business planning, financial modelling, concurrent monitoring and impact evaluation. She has over ten years of experience as a development sector practitioner and is trained in rural management.

# Social Innovations in Urban Sanitation in India

Meeting Unmet Needs

Shubhagato Dasgupta,
Kaustuv Kanti Bandyopadhyay,
Anju Dwivedi, Sumona DasGupta
and Bharti

Routledge
Taylor & Francis Group
LONDON AND NEW YORK

First published 2023
by Routledge
4 Park Square, Milton Park, Abingdon, Oxon OX14 4RN

and by Routledge
605 Third Avenue, New York, NY 10158

*Routledge is an imprint of the Taylor & Francis Group, an informa business*

*British Library Cataloguing-in-Publication Data*
A catalogue record for this book is available from the British Library

ISBN: 978-0-367-76835-5 (hbk)
ISBN: 978-1-032-05336-3 (pbk)
ISBN: 978-1-003-19710-2 (ebk)

DOI: 10.4324/9781003197102

Typeset in Sabon
by Deanta Global Publishing Services, Chennai, India

# Contents

# Figures

# Boxes

# Foreword

The history of human civilisation is a history of learning and innovations. While learning accompanied all forms of life and living since it began on planet earth, 'schools' as sites of learning were initially formalised when settlements and trades began in ancient Egypt, Mesopotamia, India or China nearly 3500 BC. Schools of that era were 'residential' (in modern terms) where living, working, learning, teaching and serving happened for youth, along with a few 'experts', variously called Gurus. They served the purpose of scaling up supply of 'skilled' persons – skilled in scriptures, recording, finance and warfare.

Around the same time, settlements began to create systems of storage of water for populations 'settled' in those sites. Early practices of formal places for defecation (and its subsequent removal/disposal) also began in such settlements. What was distinctive about the design, location and construction of such formal systems of water storage, defecation and schooling in those ancient sites (spread across settlements from Egypt to China) was the creation of contextually appropriate and adaptable (hence sustainable) solutions.

As settlements grew and urbanisation accelerated, rulers and policymakers perhaps lost sight of the core principles of creating systems essential for sustainable settlements. The present challenge for creating sustainable solutions for water and sanitation for urban settlements (now called cities and towns) is to 'recover' those core principles and to do so with different levels of technologies available to humankind today.

Sustainable solutions entail *inclusion* (works for all), *ownership* (self-governing), *networked* (organically linked to macro systems) and *ecologic* (locally appropriate use of natural/physical resources). The methodology of creating such 'socially' sustainable innovations needs to draw on a systems approach of design and implementation that combines synergistically the logic of technology with the logic of social setting and ecology. When these three logics are creatively harnessed, keeping local context in view, the solutions are innovative indeed.

This book, therefore, focuses the reader's attention on the processes of innovations that generate socially and ecologically sustainable solutions to address the needs of water and sanitation in urban settlements in India. The case studies bring practical illustrations of both the solutions produced in those diverse urban settlements but also the methodology of generating such solutions that are integrating the three sets of logics – technical, social and ecological.

Given the vast unmet needs for sustainable provision of water and sanitation services for ever-expanding urban settlements and populations in India, it is tempting to promote scaling-up through the mere multiplication of innovations found appropriate in a pilot experiment. The case studies presented in this book have many innovative features that can be thoughtfully multiplied, provided the underlying logic and processes are understood as foundational principles. Sustainable solutions for urban water, sanitation, housing and education for diverse populations and settlements must build on these distinctive innovative principles and features, but not push for a blueprint 'chip' to be 'installed' universally.

In order to be able to build on the principles and methods demonstrated in these innovations, it is important that the ecosystem of innovation is nurtured in every urban centre, not just in capital and metro locations. Facilitating the engagement of multiple stakeholders – elected leaders, officials, community organisations, professionals, investors, workers (especially sanitation workers) and vendors – in implementing such innovations is critical to promote such an ecosystem. And, as case studies have amply demonstrated, locally rooted and socially committed civil society actors can, and do, play important roles in such facilitation.

One single lesson from the pandemic now being universally acknowledged is to plant universal principles on local soil, keeping in view the local social and ecological context. It is this 'seeding' that entails innovation, not once for all, but repeatedly, everywhere, settlement by settlement, city by city.

Dr Rajesh Tandon
Founder-President
Participatory Research in Asia (PRIA)

# Acknowledgements

The Government of India launched the Swachh Bharat Mission – Urban (SBM-Urban) in 2014, which recognised the significance of citizen engagement and civil society to achieve sustainable sanitation solutions. Civil society organisations (CSOs) have been promoting contextual and sustainable innovative models to improve urban sanitation in India for decades. These innovations range from mobilising citizens, particularly from low-income communities, to generating awareness and demand services from the service providers, building community-managed systems for ensuring the sustainability of created assets, providing low-cost infrastructure solutions, organising informal sanitation workers to demand dignity and justice, generating critical knowledge and promoting collaboration and partnerships with various stakeholders including governments and private institutions to serve the unserved communities. Lessons from these social innovations, cultivated in various contexts and regions, are essential to achieve the universal sanitation goals as laid out in Sustainable Development Goals (SDGs) as well as in the national priorities.

Against this backdrop, the Centre for Policy Research (CPR) and Society for Participatory Research in Asia (PRIA) engaged in a participatory research study in partnership with several Indian CSOs and social movements which have been pioneering myriad social innovations in urban sanitation. This book is the final outcome of this research study and numerous conversations with the leadership of these organisations.

We acknowledge the support received from Bill and Melinda Gates Foundation and European Union to undertake research and organise workshops which have been critical input to this book. We gratefully acknowledge the generosity and deep insights shared by the leadership and staff members of the Centre for Urban and Regional Excellence (CURE), Centre for Science and Environment (CSE), Consortium for DEWATS Dissemination Society (CDD), Development Alternative (DA), Freshwater Action Network South Asia (FANSA), Gramalaya, Hijli Inspiration, Nidan, Safai Karmachari Andolon (SKA), Shelter Associates, Society for the Promotion of Area Resource Centres (SPARC), SWaCH and Urban Management Centre (UMC). In addition, the inspirational contributions of several other CSOs in urban sanitation have been documented and analysed in this book. We tried our best to present the social innovations pioneered by these organisations in this book; however, any omission is unintentional, and we take full responsibility.

We acknowledge the contributions of the field researchers including Anshuman Karol, Arpan De Sarkar, Kanak Tiwari, Nidhi Batra, Sukrit Nagpal and Vinika Koul who prepared the case studies of various organisations. The book would not have been possible without the contribution of Mahima Malik and Aastha Jain who helped us with background research and collating the draft manuscript. We deeply appreciate the contribution of Saon Bhattacharya who painstakingly copy-edited the manuscript. We are grateful to Shoma Choudhury for her support and guidance during the preparation and finalisation of the book chapters.

We are grateful for the support and encouragement of our colleagues from the Centre for Policy Research (CPR) and the Society for Participatory Research in Asia (PRIA). We deeply appreciate the encouragement and support from Rajesh Tandon, Founder-President of PRIA, and Yamini Aiyar, President and Chief Executive of CPR.

# Abbreviations

| | |
|---|---|
| AMRUT | Atal Mission for Rejuvenation and Urban Transformation |
| AUWS | Accelerated Urban Water Supply Programme |
| AWASH | Association of Water, Sanitation and Hygiene |
| BCC | Behaviour Change Communication |
| BMGF | Bill and Melinda Gates Foundation |
| BORDA | Bremen Overseas Research and Development Association |
| BPL | Below Poverty Line |
| BWC | Blue Water Company |
| CBOs | Community-based Organisations |
| CBUD | Capacity Building for Urban Development |
| CCS | Country Cooperation Strategy |
| CDD | Consortium for DEWATS Dissemination |
| CDEL | Capacity Development Effectiveness Ladder |
| CEPT | Centre for Environmental Planning and Technology |
| CLTS | Community-led Total Sanitation |
| CPHEEO | Central Public Health and Environmental Engineering Organisation |
| CPR | Centre for Policy Research |
| CRSP | Central Rural Sanitation Programme |
| CSE | Centre for Science and Environment |
| CSOs | Civil Society Organisations |
| CSS | Centrally Sponsored Scheme |
| CST | Cluster Septic Tank |
| CTC | Community Toilet Complexes |
| CTs/PTs | Community Toilets/Public Toilets |
| CURE | Centre for Urban and Regional Excellence |
| CWAS | Centre for Water and Sanitation |
| DA | Development Alternatives |
| DEWATS | Decentralised Wastewater Treatment Systems |
| DWWTS | Decentralised Wastewater Treatment Systems |

| | |
|---|---|
| EAWAG–SANDEC | Swiss Federal Institute for Aquatic Science and Technology – Department Sanitation, Water and Solid Waste for Development |
| ECRC | Engaged Citizen Responsive City |
| EWS | Economically Weaker Section |
| FANSA | Freshwater Action Network South Asia |
| FSSM | Faecal Sludge and Septage Management |
| FSTP | Faecal Sludge Treatment Plant |
| FYP | Five Year Plan |
| GAP | Ganga Action Plan |
| GDP | Gross Domestic Product |
| GIS | Geographic Information System |
| GIZ | Deutsche Gesellschaft für Internationale Zusammenarbeit |
| GOI | Government of India |
| GP | Gram Panchayat |
| HBM | Health Belief Model |
| HUDD | Department of Housing and Urban Development |
| IA | Implementing Agency |
| IDWSSD | International Drinking Water Supply and Sanitation Decade |
| IHHL | Individual Household Latrine |
| IHHTs | Individual Household Toilets |
| IIT | Indian Institute of Technology |
| ILCS | Integrated Low Cost Sanitation |
| ILO | International Labour Organisation |
| IMR | Infant Mortality Rate |
| JJM | Jal Jeevan Mission |
| JMP | Joint Monitoring Programme for Water Supply, Sanitation and Hygiene |
| JnNURM | Jawaharlal Nehru National Urban Renewal Mission |
| KLD | Kilolitres Per Day |
| LIG | Low Income Group |
| LNOB | Leave No One Behind |
| MC | Municipal Commissioner |
| MDGs | Millennium Development Goals |
| MGNREGS | Mahatma Gandhi National Rural Employment Guarantee Scheme |
| MLD | Million Litres Per Day |
| MOEFCC | Ministry of Environment, Forest and Climate Change |
| MOHUPA | Ministry of Housing and Urban Poverty Alleviation |
| MOUD | Ministry of Urban Development |
| MTU | Mobile Treatment Unit |
| NAC | National Advisory Council |

| | |
|---|---|
| NBA | Nirmal Bharat Abhiyan |
| NEERI | National Environmental Engineering Research Institute |
| NFSSM | National Faecal Sludge and Septage Management |
| NFSSMA | National Faecal Sludge and Septage Management Alliance |
| NGO | Non-Government Organisation |
| NGT | National Green Tribunal |
| NIUA | National Institute of Urban Affairs |
| NLCP | National Lake Conservation Plan |
| NRCP | National River Conservation Plan |
| NSKFDC | National Safai Karamchari Finance and Development Corporation |
| NSSO | National Sample Survey Office |
| NULP | National Urban Learning Platform |
| NUSP | National Urban Sanitation Policy |
| O&M | Operation and Maintenance |
| ODF | Open Defecation Free |
| OSS | On-site Sanitation |
| OUSM | Odisha Urban Sanitation Management |
| OUSP | Odisha Urban Sanitation Policy |
| OUSS | Odisha Urban Sanitation Strategy |
| OWSSB | Odisha Water Supply and Sewerage Board |
| PA | Practical Action |
| PASS | Pani Aur Swacchta Mein Sajhedari |
| PRCA | Participatory Rural Communication Appraisal |
| PMAY | Pradhan Mantri Awas Yojana |
| PPE | Personal Protective Equipment |
| PPP | Public Private Partnership |
| PRIA | Participatory Research in Asia |
| PSE | Participatory Settlement Enumeration |
| PUA | Participatory Urban Appraisal |
| R&D | Research and Development |
| RWAS | Residence Welfare Associations |
| RWH | Rainwater Harvesting |
| SA | Shelter Associates |
| SBM | Swachh Bharat Mission |
| SCBP | Sanitation Capacity Building Platform |
| SCI-FI | Scaling City Institutions for India |
| SCT | Social Cognitive Theory |
| SDA | Slum Dwellers Association |
| SDGs | Sustainable Development Goals |
| SFD | Shit Flow Diagram |
| SHE-TEAM | Sanitation and Hygiene Education – Team |
| SHF | Self-Help Federation |

| | |
|---|---|
| SHG | Self Help Group |
| SICS | Settlement Improvement Committees |
| SKA | Safai Karmachari Andolan |
| SLWM | Solid and Liquid Waste Management |
| SOP | Standard Operating Procedure |
| SPARC | Society for the Promotion of Area Resource Centres |
| SRMS | Self-Employment Scheme for Rehabilitation of Manual Scavengers |
| STP | Sewage Treatment Plant |
| SUSANA | Sustainable Sanitation Alliance |
| SWM | Solid Waste Management |
| TCC | Trichy City Corporation |
| TSC | Total Sanitation Campaign |
| TSUS | Technical Support Units |
| UCD | Urban Community Development |
| UIDSSMT | Urban Infrastructure Development Scheme for Small and Medium Towns |
| ULB | Urban Local Body |
| UMC | Urban Management Centre |
| USAID | The United States Agency for International Development |
| VIP | Ventilated Improved Pit |
| WASH | Water, Sanitation and Hygiene |
| WEDC | Water, Engineering and Development Centre |
| WSP | Water and Sanitation Program |

# Introduction

According to the Joint Monitoring Programme (JMP) of WHO and UNICEF, in 2013, 60 percent or 597 million people who practised open defecation across the world resided in India, in spite of various national sanitation programmes being in place since the 1980s. This stark statistic was possibly one of the key concerns, other than the other issues articulated by the government that propelled the Government of India to launch a programme that was deemed to be a game changer in the field of sanitation in 2014. This took the form of the much-needed Swachh Bharat Mission (SBM), which was significantly more ambitious than past programmes and aligned with the earlier National Urban Sanitation Policy (NUSP) of 2008 and the Jawaharlal Nehru National Urban Renewal Mission (JnNURM) of 2005. NUSP and JnNURM had attempted to prioritise investment for improving urban sanitation in India but had ended up generating uneven outcomes across states due to differential investments, capacities and accountability.

The SBM programme drew on elements from past programmes such as the Integrated Low-Cost Sanitation Scheme (ILCS), the Central Rural Sanitation Programme (CRSP), Total Sanitation Campaign (TSC) and Nirmal Bharat Abhiyan (NBA) but created a new canvas to instil a renewed political commitment and increased awareness among the citizenry to deal with the nation's massive sanitation challenges – essential prerequisites to the success of any large-scale programme.

As the SBM was rolled out with much vigour, the Civil Society Organisations (CSOs) who had been working on the issues of urban sanitation for decades were also encouraged by the prospect of increased access to sanitation services by the people in general and the urban poor residing in informal settlements in particular. At this time, two institutions – the Centre for Policy Research (CPR) and Participatory Research in Asia (PRIA) – were actively engaged in the discourse on accelerating the impact of the SBM by tapping not only the general enthusiasm of the prominent Indian CSOs but also utilising their decades of expertise and innovations in the urban sanitation space. This conversation among the authors from these two institutions came out of the realisation that although SBM exhibited a lot of promises, several systemic limitations might impede the realisation of its vision and objectives unless these are addressed in a systematic and time-bound manner. A critical reflection suggested that factors such as citizen participation, particularly that of the urban poor, behaviour change, institutional capacities of municipalities to foster a bottom-up planning process, and an integrated approach to scientific solid and liquid waste management would be significant factors.

The authors also deliberated that alongside governmental efforts for improving sanitation, various non-governmental institutions have experimented with innovative ideas and efforts in different regional contexts to meet the contextual needs of the community and to ensure access to safe sanitation. These experiences have the potential to hugely complement the implementation of the SBM. However, systematic documentation and critical analysis of such experimentations and their impact were missing, making these contributions less visible. This knowledge gap inspired CPR and PRIA to initiate a collaborative participatory research study with the leading CSOs working on urban sanitation in India. A joint invitation from CPR and PRIA was accepted by 12 organisations[1] to participate in this collaborative research study.

The initial focus of the study was to document the evolution of urban sanitation experimentations and interventions by each of these organisations and to draw lessons from them for mainstreaming and scaled-up practices. The preliminary documentation and analysis of organisational interventions suggested focusing on the social innovations promoted by each organisation and drawing comparative lessons around thematic clusters. From an initial literature review of the term, three features that appeared central to the idea of social innovation were (a) social innovation entailing a chain of *processes* towards finding new solutions (ideas, processes, models) to meet social needs, with technological innovation often accompanying these changes in social processes; (b) social innovations contributing to *social change* by influencing *social practices* and (c) social innovations being driven by the *intention* to produce *sustainable* and *scalable solutions* derived from local contexts to address societal issues.

This renewed focus on social innovations stimulated CPR and PRIA to convene a dialogue with research participants as well as other researchers and practitioners working on urban sanitation. The idea of a multistakeholder conference germinated through numerous conversations, and finally a national conference, Social Innovations for Improving Urban Sanitation: Lessons for Scaling-Up, was held in December 2016. All the participating organisations in the research study contributed to highlighting the multifaceted social innovations within the broad framework described above. The post-conference deliberations among the authors brought out three important facets, which shaped the content and arrangement of this book.

First, in most organisational examples, the idea of social innovations came out of a well-identified 'unmet need', primarily of the marginalised communities but also that of the programme implementers (government and non-government), policy researchers as well as policymakers. Second, the theoretic construct of social innovation needed practical illustrations, drawing lessons from case studies. This could be better achieved through an inductive approach rather than a deductive one. Third, the rich repository of social innovations fostered by the CSOs held enormous potential to address some of the most vexing problems plaguing the goal of sanitation for all in the Indian urban landscape, if these were scaled up. This required a systematisation of knowledge and constructive, evidence-based engagement among the community, researchers, CSOs and policymakers alike.

These insights generated over the deliberations at the national conference where the research findings were discussed and presented were the inspiration behind the book, *Social Innovations in Urban Sanitation from India: Meeting Unmet Needs*. The book discusses the social innovations in the urban sanitation sector, facilitated by several Indian CSOs. The idea of social innovation as 'new ideas that meet unmet needs' typically operates across organisational and sectoral boundaries and involves a coming together of existing elements that link ideas, people, finance and power. The book argues that social innovations in urban sanitation programmes developed and supported by CSOs need to have certain characteristics – such as building effective alliances, demanding services, strengthening community-managed systems, designing low-cost solutions, organising informal sanitation workers and serving marginalised communities – to be able to influence public policy. The authors present the contours of an ecosystem for social innovations in urban sanitation that keep communities and people as active participants in the process of change and remain locally and contextually sensitive even as these innovations are standardised and scaled up.

The enormity of the sanitation challenge and the absence of literature on urban sanitation from a social innovation perspective make this book particularly relevant now. While the SBM has made laudable progress to address this, what has not yet received adequate attention is the ongoing work of many CSOs and people's movements that have experimented with smaller, innovative ideas with the potential to be scaled up to meet community needs in urban sanitation. Innovations have ranged from providing low-cost infrastructure solutions, demanding services from service providers by mobilising citizens, building and strengthening community-managed systems for ensuring the sustainability of created assets, organising informal sanitation workers to demand dignity and justice, and promoting and building collaboration and partnerships with various stakeholders, including government and private agencies to serve marginalised communities. In turning the searchlights on such initiatives in urban sanitation by drawing on multiple case studies across India, this book aims to mine lessons from on-ground solutions in urban sanitation and indicate how to scale them up and allow them to inform national policymaking.

Most of the available literature on urban sanitation in India is data-heavy with an emphasis on rural sanitation against urban sanitation, which is the focus of this book. Most of these books explore specific aspects of sanitation from a single perspective, such as only the legal or economic aspect (pricing) of basic services. The role of the community in making such technical solutions successful is rarely discussed in such literature. This book addresses this critical gap by addressing how innovative solutions are created, adopted and become embedded in a sociocultural context to achieve the desired outcome of sanitation for all.

Earlier works often present detailed individual case studies of how city administrators/managers found strategies to affect change at the city level. But the specificities of a local-level solution hide the generalities that policymakers need to scale up innovative solutions to create any significant impact across the country. This book helps fill this gap by mining lessons from on-ground solutions and translating them into scalable, national-level policymaking.

The significance of this book comes from how it approaches the analysis of urban sanitation through the lens of social innovation, turning the searchlights on how existing (rather than new) elements related to sanitation come together innovatively, and how community-level sanitation practices can cut across organisational, sectoral and disciplinary boundaries, setting in motion a set of new relationships between previously disjointed individuals and groups. This in turn carries the potential to trigger off innovations. It is the novelty of this lens that enables readers to see a very different picture of the urban sanitation arena in India offering a glimpse of what happens where change makers innovate to 'meet unmet needs' by placing the community at the heart of the process and enabling their participation in solving the huge challenge of providing inclusive urban sanitation.

Methodologically the book also breaks new grounds by researching 13 CSOs that have worked innovatively on urban sanitation across the country and then drawing on the corpus of primary data sourced from these case studies for analysis. This methodology enables the narratives in this book to speak from the perspective of the poor and marginalised with whom the CSOs included in the case studies have worked closely. The new corpus of evidence also helps to indicate how policies and programmes can become more inclusive in design and implementation; and in doing so, this book speaks to a broader, larger audience across South Asia and the developing Global South.

This book seeks to be a game changer because by bringing a new perspective to the study of urban sanitation in India, it suggests a whole new way in which the issue can be approached. Keeping in mind the rationale behind this book, it has been organised into nine chapters following this introductory chapter.

The first chapter, 'Urban Sanitation Landscape in India: Setting the Context', draws on the recent evolution of India's sanitation policy. It demonstrates how sanitation policies in the past have evolved through a process of social innovation. Such innovative approaches can play a significant role in contributing to India's aspiration to meet the global agenda of Sustainable Development Goal 6 (SDG 6) on clean water and sanitation. Presenting an evolutionary perspective through the Five-Year Plans, the chapter marks the milestones influencing and impacting the sanitation landscape since 1980. Illustrating the urban sanitation journey, the chapter critically reflects upon the challenges in this sector. These include building capacities of all stakeholders; sustained access and functionality of the sanitation infrastructure; safe and scientific solid waste, faecal sludge and septage management; complete prohibition of manual scavenging; and reaching the most marginalised. In light of these challenges, this chapter argues for a new framework that can provide ways for CSOs, community-based organisations (CBOs) and the government to move beyond conventional solutions and catalyse various changes – social, cultural and technological. This chapter aims to set the tone and underscore the need to critically analyse sanitation components and amplify the voices of the marginalised to bring social and policy change.

Following this historical analysis of the evolution of innovative practices in urban sanitation, the second chapter, 'Social Innovation in Urban Sanitation: Experiences from India', unpacks the concept of social innovation in more detail. Drawing on the literature on social innovations from the 1990s onwards, it applies the conceptual frameworks to understand the changes being made in the Indian urban sanitation context. In doing so, it draws extensively on specific case studies from across the country where experiments and interventions in urban sanitation have placed households and communities at the heart. It begins by arriving at a working definition of the term social innovation and then delves into different components of these innovations in the context of urban sanitation in India. To do this, it examines community-based innovations in urban sanitation by a host of CSOs. This chapter, therefore, describes how social innovations adapt existing technologies to meet unmet needs by introducing green technology to decentralised wastewater management or encouraging home-based solutions to people's needs for toilets through improvised ideas field-tested in rural sanitation for urban use (such as the construction of leach pit toilets). It draws attention to strategies, methods and tools to organise the unorganised communities to amplify their voices to access urban sanitation services and realise their rights and dignity. It highlights how an organisation created a movement to abolish manual scavenging by restoring dignity, safety and health to the core of their social innovation on urban sanitation. The chapter also touches on social innovations such as providing a chain of deliverables in the sanitation sector and organising hawkers and vendors to be at the forefront of urban sanitation issues.

The subsequent chapters then move on to focus on the different dimensions of social innovation.

The third chapter, 'Organisation Building for Inclusive Urban Sanitation: Organising the Unorganised', focuses on mobilising the unorganised sector in urban sanitation by drawing on the key tenets of social innovations as new ways of doing things that change the direction of social change while improving the quality of life, especially for the marginalised population. The chapter centres on building organisations for the poor and marginalised to meet the unmet needs of sanitation and bring about social transformation by mobilising the collective voices of people in a way that they become part of the solution. Strengthening community organisations, facilitating communication channels between privileged and non-privileged citizens, and creating participatory and democratic forums are the key elements in this category of social innovations. It highlights the necessity to connect people with governments and other stakeholders in civil society to create intersectionality in organisation building, which is critical to social innovation in urban sanitation. The chapter illustrates the strategies adopted by the CSOs for strengthening collective demand through community platforms leading to collective strength, voice, strategy and leadership of the economically disadvantaged and the vulnerable in becoming a part of the movement for urban sanitation. It demonstrates the impact of organisation building in improving the quality of life of marginalised people by improving their access to services, ensuring safety and justice and making governance institutions more accountable and transparent by examining specific cases in the arena of urban sanitation.

This book then goes on to analyse the impact of such organisation building in terms of behaviour change. The fourth chapter, 'Sustainable Behaviour Change in Community', explores various innovations primarily facilitated by the CSOs in urban sanitation spaces to encourage behaviour change among communities and other stakeholders. Development communication has always remained a powerful approach for reaching out to people with messages and information so that attitudinal and behaviour change can be affected to bring desired social change. This understanding prompted the Swachh Bharat Mission – Urban (SBM-U) and the National Policy on Faecal Sludge and Septage Management (FSSM) to emphasise awareness generation and behaviour change campaigns acknowledging that the technological innovations and investments in infrastructure can only sustain with strategic communication approaches. However, the chapter makes a distinction between promoting individual behavioural change and collective behavioural change. The former is deeply associated with broader social change that can mobilise public action for policy changes. It showcases that whenever participatory communication approaches are adopted, communication takes the form of dialogue to identify a problem, reflect and articulate it, analyse it and come up with a solution for it. Hence, participatory communication is a process of social change and a key element of social innovation. As demonstrated through case studies, awareness generation and enhanced knowledge and information lead to greater accountability and improved service delivery due to greater demand from the community. Greater knowledge of the use of toilets and improved health of onsite sanitation systems created demand on urban local bodies to provide quick and efficient services of timely desludging of onsite sanitation systems and creating decentralised systems for faecal sludge management.

Integral to this behaviour change is raising a new public consciousness around sanitation work. The fifth chapter, 'Sanitation Work and Workers: Prioritising Issues of Rights, Dignity and Safety', analyses host innovations by the CSOs, which have enabled access to the rights and dignity of sanitation workers and reduced the drudgery of their work. It traces the evolution of laws, policies and programmes directed at ameliorating the dismal condition of sanitation workers, particularly manual scavengers, while pointing to the problem of lackadaisical implementation and lack of accountability of public institutions. Not only is the very nature of sanitation work hazardous, but the working conditions of sanitation workers in India are also rendered extremely precarious because of their inescapable association with the caste system. This links sanitation as the sole concern of the scheduled castes, particularly the Valmiki community. Adding another layer of complexity is the gender fault line with women sanitation workers living and working under the double burden of labour (wage earners as well as household caregivers). The case exemplars highlight the efforts to mobilise sanitation workers and public opinion against manual scavenging, the gender dimension of sanitation work and the use of research from an equity and inclusive lens to connect policymakers and organisations of sanitation workers by highlighting the precarious working conditions of such workers and their lack of access to various government programmes and schemes. This chapter also suggests policy recommendations for effective safety measures, better dignity and access to rights for sanitation workers.

The sixth chapter, 'Innovative Technology: Connecting the Disconnect', highlights that to the extent that every technological innovation is a response to a social problem, it constitutes a social action in and of itself. Undoubtedly, there is a critical role played by technology in meeting unmet human needs, which lies at the heart of the idea of social innovation. However, all too often the full impact of technology is lost because it is viewed in isolation and attributed as the sole factor responsible for human progress. The chapter demonstrates how the impact of technology is enhanced when it is linked with 'pro-poor' innovations. It submits that when appropriate technologies are linked with specific needs of the community – in this case, the sanitation needs of the urban poor and other marginalised groups – the impact of that technology is multiplied. When a mutually reinforcing relationship is established between technical innovation and social needs, the former is much more likely to be accepted and diffused; and to that extent its full potential is realised. The chapter argues that when technology is placed on a pedestal and uses terminology that is beyond the understanding of the community whose interests it is supposed to serve, it can be alienating. Therefore, unpacking technological solutions is critical for the community of users to understand, invest in and participate in the process of finding innovative solutions for urban sanitation.

The seventh chapter, 'Multistakeholder Capacity Building for Inclusive Urban Sanitation', examines innovative practices for capacity building of multiple stakeholders in urban sanitation. Capacity is the ability of an entity to achieve its mission or mandate; and enhancing it requires strengthening its intellectual, institutional and resource base. This chapter delineates three levels of capacity building – (a) at the individual level, with leadership and human resources; (b) at the institutional level, with organisational strategy, structure, technology, processes and culture and (c) at the sectoral level, with enabling laws, policies and other external environments. It argues that for social innovations in the urban sanitation sector to be successful, a well-strategised capacity-building effort for relevant stakeholders needs to be in place to address capacities in all areas and at all levels. The SBM and Atal Mission for Rejuvenation and Urban Transformation (AMRUT), the coveted programmes of the Central Government on urban water and sanitation, provide critical resources to local municipalities for programme implementation. However, the required capacities of municipalities for designing, planning, implementing, monitoring and assessing the programmes sustainably and inclusively are far from adequate. The urban sanitation programme that works for all in the city across socio-economic classes and all genders would require engagement by multiple stakeholders. Since there has been very little precedent of multistakeholder engagement in a city context, the capacities of all stakeholders need to be enhanced to make sanitation services more inclusive. For this, capacity-building interventions must be planned and implemented for state and local governance institutions, civil society and citizens' organisations as well as private institutions. This chapter discusses the innovative practices of building capacities of low-income communities, municipalities and other stakeholders on participatory planning, septage management, municipal solid waste management, planning and designing of decentralised wastewater treatment, water-sensitive urban design and planning, using both classroom and field-based learning methods.

Whether it is exploring new horizons in technology to further the goal of achieving urban sanitation for all, or creating awareness among people to accept such technological changes and change their behaviour as a result, the role of research and advocacy becomes critical. Consequently, the eighth chapter, 'Urban Sanitation: Policy Research and Advocacy', describes how community action and institutional action can be synergised through research and advocacy so that, equipped with necessary information and ideas of what is feasible at the community level, it becomes easier for people to demand accountability in the arena of urban sanitation as well as scale up local initiatives. The chapter deals with two central questions. First, what kind of research and knowledge sharing is needed to create enabling conditions for social innovations in urban sanitation to take off at the community level and identify the concurrent issues that allow for community-level innovations to be scaled up through public policy? And second, what kind of awareness campaigns, research sharing and advocacy is needed to make these innovations socially impactful once they take off? This chapter draws on specific research and advocacy tools used by CSOs working at the community level in the urban sanitation sector. It illustrates such efforts of CSOs to understand the sociocultural aspects of urban sanitation and cultural reasons for open defecation, highlighting the inadequacy of knowledge, information and awareness among the community; non-networked sanitation systems and the importance of implementing such models to address sanitation challenges in India; and the critical role of evidence-based research and policy advocacy in spreading its basic social innovation message for viewing sanitation as a social participatory issue that is intrinsically linked with water management. It also analyses the impact of policy-level dialogues convened by some of the CSOs while leveraging existing relationships with marginalised communities and sanitation workers.

The final chapter, Conclusion, concludes by highlighting the nature of social innovations fostered by the CSOs in the urban sanitation spaces while suggesting some critical factors for mainstreaming and scaling up these innovations. The book has drawn attention to recent innovative practices in urban sanitation that citizens have initiated, catalysed by CSOs to meet their unmet needs when state institutions and market mechanics have fallen short of fulfilling their requirements. Our primary finding has been that it is the CSOs that have helped empower marginalised communities to access urban sanitation services, provided institutional frameworks of solidarity to accompany technological innovations, transformed social relations and encouraged new forms of governance and community participation. It highlights social innovations in urban sanitation as transformative in nature as they not only find solutions to complex problems but also aim to generate change within the institutional ecosystem responsible for solving those problems by bringing adequate policy focus through research, advocacy and strengthening capacities of all stakeholders. Social innovations are also local and context-specific, as gleaned through various CSO-led interventions described in this book, but have the potential to disseminate and scale up by receiving policy focus and being diffused to the contexts facing similar intractable challenges and unmet needs.

Social innovation is a continuous process as new unmet needs emerge with time. Such innovations can help mitigate some intractable problems; but new challenges emerge, thus promoting social innovations to grow and adapt to meet the unfulfilled needs of the people. New paradigms for improving urban sanitation systems are already becoming visible. The challenges emerging from climate change are bringing sanitation systems in many well-served communities at risk. Coastal communities and flood and drought-prone areas are increasingly facing sanitation challenges that were not considered earlier. Similarly, the demand for improving sanitation services across geographies in rapidly urbanising contexts in developing countries also has to consider issues not considered in the past. Other issues are also expected to emerge. Social innovations, therefore, remain critical to addressing future emerging challenges and need support to thrive and survive. Social innovations need appropriate conditions to take roots, such as strong leadership and vision by social innovators, partnerships and alliances, enhanced capacities of institutions to respond to intractable problems, empowerment of communities and the most marginalised to gain a voice to articulate their unmet needs and demand accountability from the institutions of governance. This book provides evidence of the critical role that CSOs and the social innovations championed by them have played in the past and continue to play in the current march towards global, safely managed sanitation, alongside governments taking more responsibility and increasing support to the sector. It is hoped that this book will also reignite a constructive discussion on how all stakeholders could contribute to creating a more robust ecosystem for social innovation and the critical role that CSOs need to continue to play in the sector.

## Note

1 Centre for Science and Environment (CSE), Centre for Urban and Regional Excellence (CURE), Consortium for DEWATS Dissemination Society (CDD), Development Alternatives, Freshwater Action Network South Asia (FANSA), Gramalaya, Nidan, Safai Karmachari Andolon (SKA), Shelter Associates, Society for the Promotion of Area Resource Centres (SPARC), SWaCH Cooperatives and Urban Management Centre (UMC).

# 1 Urban Sanitation Landscape in India
## Setting the Context

## 1. INTRODUCTION

Urban sanitation in modern India remains a distressing problem. Despite certain significant advancements, there remain numerous issues and concerns to address. Modern urban sanitation first transformed public health and urban life in the 19th century in Western Europe and North America. However, in South Asia, including India, during the colonial 19th century and the first half of the 20th century, much of the state's public efforts were targeted at ensuring public health improvements through water and sewerage projects in locations where the colonial British and the elite resided, as well as at ensuring the health of the army, at the cost of extending improved services to the local population living in older cities and villages. Post-independence, while some efforts to improve conditions were taken up in an era of nation-building, neither they were of adequate scale nor was the geographic bias adequately addressed (Chaplin, 2011). It was during 1980–1990 that the International Drinking Water Supply and Sanitation Decade (IDWSSD) was launched at a global level, and India responded through the launch of large-scale programmes such as Integrated Low-Cost Sanitation (ILCS) in 1981, Ganga Action Plan (GAP) in 1985 and Central Rural Sanitation Programme (CRSP) in 1986. This chapter reviews the evolution of urban sanitation and sanitation policies in independent India, to provide a context to the sanitation efforts that civil society organisations (CSOs) have been involved in.

After close to two generations of sanitation investments since the 1980s by both private households and governments, in 2011, more than 50 percent of the population in India practised open defecation (OD), while 3 percent depended on public toilets (PTs) and 47 percent had access to an in-house latrine (IHL) (Census, 2011). During the 12th Five-Year Plan (FYP), the last of India's Five-Year Plans, the Swachh Bharat Mission (SBM) was launched as the flagship project to accelerate efforts towards universal sanitation coverage and drive sanitation investments across rural and urban areas. This was followed by the Atal Mission for Rejuvenation and Urban Transformation (AMRUT) and Smart City Mission in 2015 to accentuate efforts and investments in urban infrastructure, including that of sanitation

DOI: 10.4324/9781003197102-1

in larger cities. Since 2014, India has witnessed significant strides in basic sanitation improvements in urban and rural areas. On 2 October 2019, the 150th birth anniversary of the Father of the Nation, Mahatma Gandhi, the Government of India announced that all rural households had access to basic safe sanitation and that all villages had declared themselves Open Defecation Free (ODF). While there is evidence that this claim may have been an overestimation, all scholars across the board agree that over the past few years the access to and use of toilets have increased rapidly.

This chapter sets the context and presents an analysis of the recent state of urban sanitation in India. It then discusses government policies from an evolutionary perspective through successive Five-Year Plans. The chapter covers some of the important milestones influencing and impacting sanitation in India since 1980 and the role of global water and sanitation-focused development institutions, from the start of the IDWSSD. Special reference is made to water and sanitation projects driven by CSOs and public programmes initiated by governments in search of new innovative approaches and technologies for scaling up sanitation. Early examples of service delivery and technology innovations include the development of the ventilated improved pit (VIP), the twin pit composting latrine and the operational model for pay-and-use community toilets. Other institutional innovations included the creation of water and sanitation parastatal bodies, strengthening of state and national environment protection agencies, and involvement of new participatory models such as the Community-Led Total Sanitation model, sanitation marketing models, targeted behaviour change campaigns and laws to support the health and dignity challenges of sanitation workers. The chapter also discusses these new participatory models as social innovations that generated institutional change. Recent innovations around models for city-wide faecal sludge management systems are also discussed. Many of these innovations were piloted through CSO action and are now institutionalised in government sanitation policies and programmes, demonstrating the co-dependencies between social innovations and meeting unmet needs at scale, in a rapidly changing context.

## 2. SANITATION STATUS IN CONTEMPORARY INDIA

India had a total population of 1.2 billion in 2011, with 833 million living in rural and 377 million in urban India (Census, 2011). It was the second most populous country in 2011, with an estimated urban population set to increase by 221 million by 2031, which is almost equal to the population of Brazil or Indonesia. The scale of the sanitation problem in India, even after achieving ODF status, is enormous. Prioritising sanitation in India is a global as well as a national necessity, as improvement in its sanitation situation is imperative for improving global access to sanitation and public health. In 2011, when the last census was conducted in India, IHLs in rural areas had increased from a mere 1 percent in 1981 to just above 31 percent, and defecation in the open (OD) was still practised by 67 percent of the population. In urban areas, even when 81 percent had IHLs, 6 percent had access to PTs and 13 percent practised OD, urban India still led 52 percent of the world's urban OD (Figure 1.1) (Census, 2011).

While there has been under-investment in the urban sanitation sector, generally there are significant social institutions and behavioural issues too that have constrained the population at large from investing in basic sanitation infrastructure of toilets within their homes. A survey on Sanitation Quality, Use, Access and Trends (SQUAT Survey, 2014) across five states in rural India revealed that over 40 percent of households with a working latrine had at least one member who defecated in the open. Forty-seven percent of those who defecated in the open said they did so because it was pleasant, comfortable or convenient. The revealed preference for OD is not entirely a rural phenomenon and can be observed in urban India too, especially in numerous small and medium towns that make up India's urban system. The behavioural preferences of a large proportion of the population allude to the fact that merely providing latrine 'access' without promoting latrine use is unlikely to reduce OD. The latrines are considered 'unclean'. The concept of sanitation and hygiene is closely related to the perceptions of pollution, dirt, filth and cleanliness (Smith, 2007). People have culturally patterned beliefs about what is clean and what is unclean, what is pure and what is polluting, and it is this cultural context that determines behaviour patterns (Bauman, 1998). Such values are of immense importance for how sanitation can be organised and upheld in communities across India, where it is associated with behaviours and practices like defecating outside and away from the house in an attempt to keep the house 'pure' and away from 'polluting' activities like defecation. This social institutional understanding

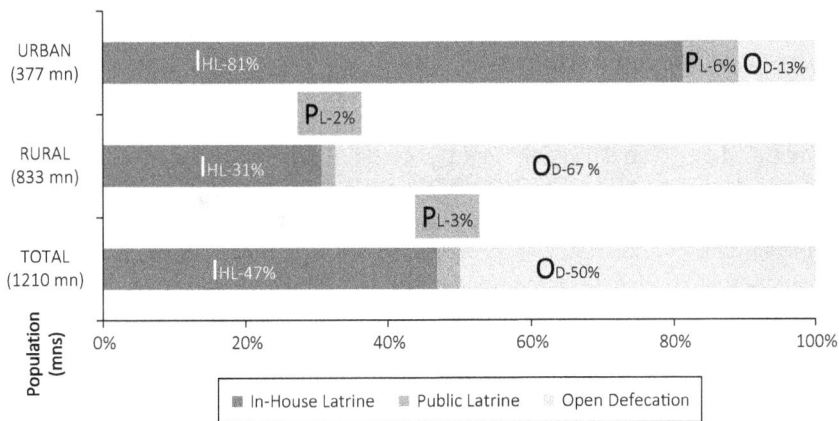

*Figure 1.1* Access to toilets. Source: Census of India, 2011

has been identified to be a significant barrier to the access and use of in-house toilets among more traditional communities in the country.

Despite these constraints, as per the latest figures from the SBM (Urban) initiative, 58,46,107 individual toilets have been built in urban areas – exclusive of 4,99,006 community and public toilets. Additionally, 4,303 cities were declared ODF as on 1 October 2019 (Swachh Bharat Mission Urban, Ministry of Housing and Urban Affairs, 2019). Data from SBM (Rural) shows that as on 1 October 2019, 699 districts had declared themselves as ODF, which effectively means that India is now ODF as far as self-declaration is concerned (Swachh Bharat Mission Gramin, Ministry of Jal Shakti, 2019). How soon will all these districts be verified as ODF is something that remains to be seen. While OD has remained a significant challenge, ensuring its eradication would only be a first step in solving the sanitation crisis that India is currently facing. A holistic approach that covers the entire sanitation value chain has been articulated by scholars and experts alike, to make sure that sanitation systems cover both public health and environmental pollution problems. This would include ensuring regular operations and maintenance (O&M) of the constructed toilets, along with proper septage and sewerage infrastructure as well as management and change in behavioural attitudes of end-users across each element of the sanitation value chain.

## 3. KEY CHARACTERISTICS OF INDIA'S URBAN SANITATION CHALLENGE

### *Change in urban open defecation practices is not dependent on economic factors alone*

In a cross-country comparison over time, it is evident that improvement in sanitation and reduction of open defecation is not completely explained by economic status and progress alone in India and elsewhere. This characteristic of sanitation can be witnessed when sanitation and per capita improvements are compared across 11 countries – viz., Ghana, Ethiopia, Mozambique, Nigeria, Indonesia, Nepal, India, Vietnam, Bangladesh, Sri Lanka and Peru. In 1990, these 11 countries led more than 65 percent of the world's urban OD (WHO/UNICEF JMP, 2013). Figure 1.2 reveals that sanitation improvement in these nations, alongside their per capita GDP improvement over the last two decades (1990–2011), had not evenly affected the reduction in OD. In Vietnam, the urban OD level had reduced substantially from 20.3 percent to 0 percent, with per capita GDP and OD levels similar to those of India in 1990. The urban OD levels of Ethiopia, Nepal and Mozambique had reduced significantly despite any major improvement in their GDP; while Indonesia's GDP per capita had increased significantly but its reported reduction of urban OD was less significant. India, a country with the largest population practising OD in urban areas, showed

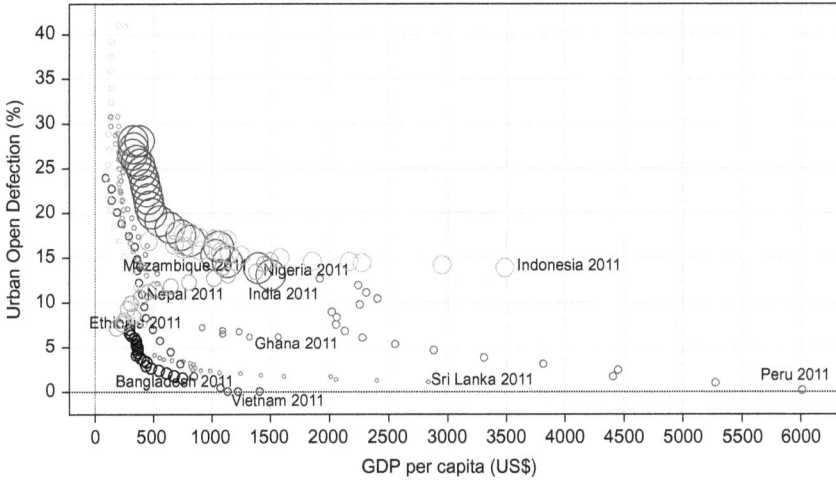

*Figure 1.2* Open defecation (urban) by GDP (1990–2011). Source: WHO and UNICEF, 2013; World Bank, 2013a

improvement in reducing OD levels with an increase in GDP. Peru managed to reduce its OD level to 0 percent and improved its economy ahead of all the other countries. By 2011, Bangladesh, the eighth most densely populated country (World Bank, 2011), Ghana and Sri Lanka also reduced their OD levels to 0.6 percent, 7.3 percent and 1.1 percent, respectively, with Sri Lanka witnessing the highest growth in per capita GDP during this period. Nigeria was a clear outlier in this trend, reporting rising urban OD levels even with an increase in per capita GDP. Although the total population practising OD in urban areas decreased from 1,34,456 in 1990 to 1,04,366 in 2011 (WHO and UNICEF, 2013), there was still a long way to go.

### Strong linkages between open defecation and infant mortality rates (IMR) across most countries, including India

The close linkage between health and sanitation is shown in Figure 1.3. The spread of disease through the faecal–oral chain has been attributed as a major cause of high IMR (WHO and UNICEF, 2013). Access to sanitation facilities improves the well-being of children. Sanitation systems form a barrier against the spread of diseases caused by pathogens and other organisms present in human excreta. Of the countries in this database, 10 of the 11 countries mapped in Figure 1.3 show a positive correlation between a reduction in urban OD levels and a simultaneous decrease in IMR.

Ethiopia, Mozambique and India had quickly reduced their urban OD levels along with their IMR, with Ethiopia showing the fastest reduction

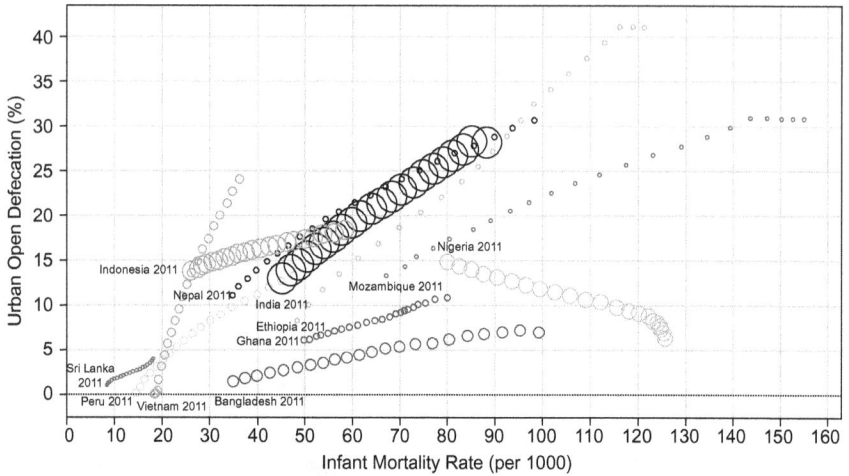

*Figure 1.3* Urban open defecation and infant mortality rate (1990–2011). Source: WHO and UNICEF, 2013; World Bank, 2013

rate. Indonesia, Nepal and Ghana had sharply reduced their IMR like India, but their urban OD had not fallen as sharply. Vietnam and Peru had reduced OD to 0 percent, and Sri Lanka too had reduced its OD and IMR levels. Nigeria was the outlier in this trend. Its urban OD level had gone up despite a decrease in IMR.

### High level of state disparities in urban sanitation in India

Urban OD levels across states in India vary widely, showing highly uneven development. On tracking urban OD against the state GDP per capita, Figure 1.4 shows three clear clusters. First, smaller states with higher income have lower OD levels. Second, large-sized states have OD rates similar to that of India's average OD; and third, medium-sized states with lower urbanisation levels have the highest OD. For instance, the maximum urban OD in India is seen in Chhattisgarh, Odisha, Jharkhand, Bihar and Madhya Pradesh.

### Toilet penetration and OD trends across city sizes in India reveal that smaller cities have disproportionately high OD levels

As shown in Figure 1.5, smaller cities lag behind larger cities in both access to IHLs and the share of the population practising OD. Class IA and IB cities with a population of 1–5 million have a greater number of toilets available for their urban population. Access to IHLs in smaller, Class II and IV cities and towns with a population below 100,000 is lower

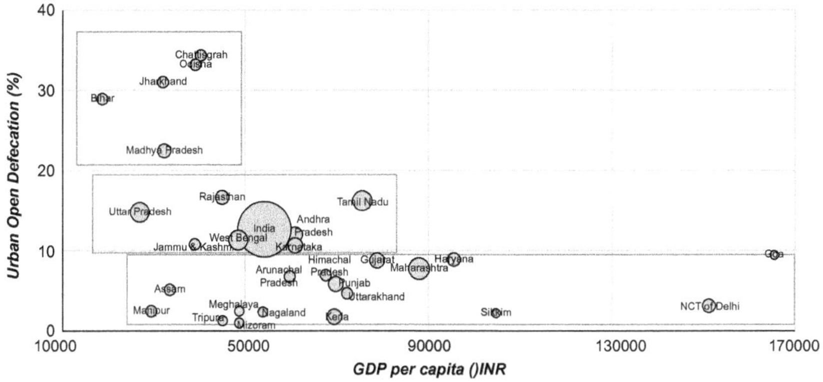

*Figure 1.4* GDP per capita and urban OD share across states. Source: Census of India, 2011

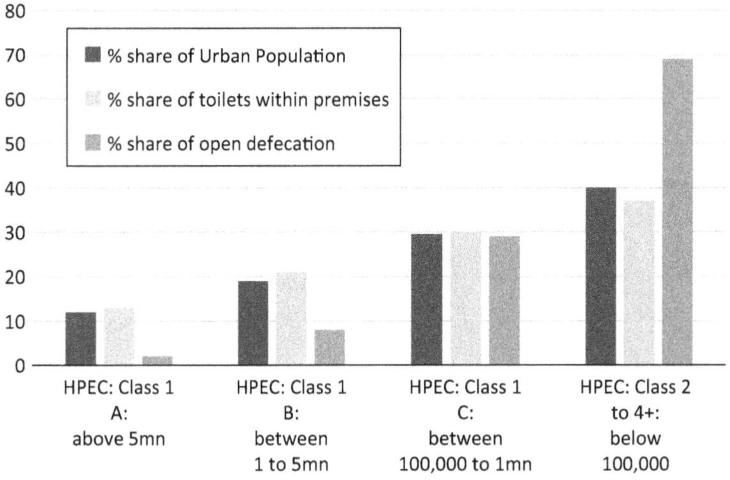

*Figure 1.5* Sanitation trend by city size. Source: Census of India, 2011

than that of larger cities. As a result, quite high OD levels are reported in these small towns. As per Census 2011, the share of OD from small towns (population below 100,000) stood at 80 percent of the total OD in urban India, which is almost twice the share of the population of these towns. Against this trend, the largest cities account for only 1 percent of the total OD in urban areas, which is close to 10 percent of India's total urban population.

## OD *is not restricted to slums alone, higher slum and non-slum* OD *noted in less urbanised states*

Figure 1.5 points towards another phenomenon, which is usually not highlighted – Urban Non-Slum Open defecation. It needs to be noted that the population practising OD does not live in informal settlements alone, as the general perception goes. There is enough evidence to show that residents of non-slum areas practise OD as well. Odisha, Chhattisgarh, Jharkhand, Bihar and Madhya Pradesh are home to the highest proportion of residents from both informal and formal settlements practising OD in urban India. Figure 1.6 also reveals that in higher urbanised states like Karnataka, Tamil Nadu and Maharashtra, the difference between OD practised in informal and formal settlements is also as varied as that in low urbanised states.

## *Inadequate capacities for wastewater and septage treatment across Indian cities*

Inadequate treatment of domestic wastewater accounts for 75 percent (Ministry of Urban Development, 2008) of water pollution. Increasing population density, the constraint of space, lack of sewage pipe connections and functional sewerage treatment plants (STPs) have led to continued large dependence on on-site sanitation facilities such as septic tanks. It is estimated that Class I and II cities and towns alone generate 72,368 MLD of sewage, while their urban local bodies (ULBs) have a capacity to treat 36,668 MLD, which is only 50 percent of the generated sewage (Central Pollution Control Board, 2021). The capacities in smaller towns are even less in terms of the proportion of wastewater collected by STPs. Simultaneously, the limited but growing capacity of faecal sludge treatment plants in the country means that much of the waste from toilets is discharged untreated into the environment too.

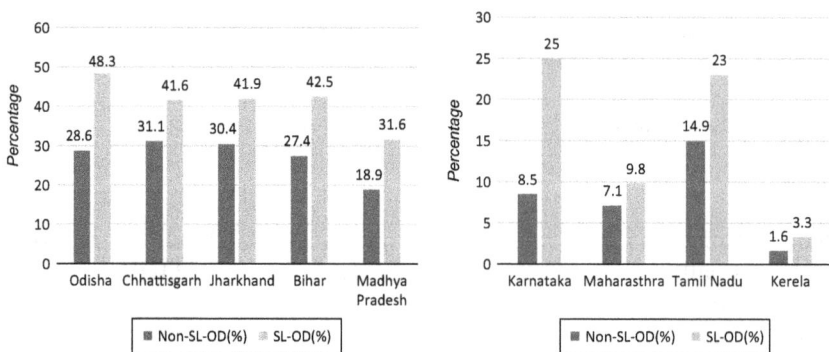

*Figure 1.6* OD in informal and formal settlements (2011). Source: Census of India, 2011

## 4. COLLABORATIVE ENDEAVOURS BY INTERNATIONAL DEVELOPMENT PARTNERS ON SANITATION

In the 1970s, sanitation in developing countries emerged as a new development objective for international development aid institutions (Black & Fawcett, 2008). Research studies backed the new realisation as a global public health concern that could not be tackled if the developing world did not have a safe public health infrastructure. A major impetus for the early research and sanitation projects that the multilateral development institutions initiated in the 1970s came from the United Nations (UN) declaring the decade between 1980 and 1990 as the International Drinking Water Supply and Sanitation Decade. This declaration was backed by the UN and supported by a large number of countries including India. This declaration also meant that all developing countries prioritised water and sanitation improvement efforts. While water supply got more attention than sanitation during this period, countries also initiated sanitation programmes. In India, new sanitation programmes were taken up at the national level and included the ILCS initiative focused on urban areas and the CRSP. In India, in support of the new environmental pollution protection policies initiated in the 1970s, large new sanitation programmes to control environmental pollution were also imitated. Primary among these was the GAP, set up to control wastewater pollution from cities along the Ganga river basin. The GAP programme initiated a large number of sewerage and STP projects in the cities by the Ganga river. During this decade, sanitation became a subject of national priority in India.

The IDWSSD also led to the creation of a new set of global water and sanitation technical assistance programmes, including the Water and Sanitation Collaborative Council, the WaterAid and the Water and Sanitation Program (initially housed under the United Nations Development Programme (UNDP) and later under the World Bank). In India, these development partners were instrumental in bringing about a substantial change at the ground level, while affecting the national policy outlook. These institutions engaged both with governments for policy formulation and infrastructure investment programmes and with CSOs to pilot innovative social and technology projects.

One of the earliest development partners in sanitation was UNICEF, which had been active in the field since 1966. While initially most of its efforts were in rural sanitation, it increased its attention to the issue of Water Sanitation and Hygiene (WASH) in urban areas too. UNICEF's key initiatives include advocating WASH through data, evidence, information and knowledge, stimulating demand, adopting community approaches to eliminate open defecation and improving children's learning environment by ensuring access to sanitation facilities and hygiene practices in schools.

Another organisation that has been active for more than three decades in India is UNDP. The UNDP Global Project (1980) in India assisted and promoted the installation of water-seal latrines in 110 towns across seven states (Planning Commission: 6th FYP, 1981). Pilot projects were taken up in these states to provide low-cost water-seal latrines with on-site disposal of human waste. Another important international development partner promoted by the UNDP and the World Bank in the field of sanitation services was the Water and Sanitation Program (WSP). WSP started work in India in the 1980s soon after it was established and focused on rural water innovations but soon moved to sanitation as well as to working in urban areas. In the 2000s, it moved its focus to support large-scale institutional reform agendas in India to aid the government in making services work for the poor within limited budgetary resources. At this stage, it also advocated urban water and sanitation through fiscal reforms that push for the decentralisation and improved sustainability of water supply and sanitation interventions.

Besides the two major UN organisations, WaterAid was set up in 1986 as an international non-governmental development implementation organisation raising funds from donor governments to support social and technological innovation in water and sanitation in developing countries. With its focus on drinking water security, rural and urban sanitation, and WASH in health and nutrition, WaterAid has since been working with a host of CSOs across the developing world, including in India.

The World Bank and the Asian Development Bank (ADB) have remained other important partners of the Indian government since the 1970s in funding for key national policy initiatives. Recently, the World Bank has been supporting the SBM (Rural) programme with a US$1.5 billion loan for SBM aimed at ending the practice of open defecation by 2019. The World Health Organisation (WHO) has led the way across development partners in providing health-based guidelines relating to the importance of clean water and proper sanitation in urban and rural areas through the Country Cooperation Strategy (CCS) under its Health of Mothers and Children priority sector. CCS was brought out in 2017. The WHO–UNICEF Joint Monitoring Programme (JMP), affiliated with UN-Water, was established in 1990. It built on earlier monitoring activities carried out by WHO since the 1960s. The JMP's objectives are to provide regular global reports on drinking water and sanitation coverage to facilitate sector planning and management, to support countries in their efforts to improve their monitoring systems and to provide information for advocacy.

While these international organisations were part of a global movement to improve water and sanitation in developing countries, after the IDWSSD, another boost from the global governance institutions came in 2000, with the UN setting up the Millennium Development Goals (MDGs) as a multilaterally negotiated set of universal and global development goals to be achieved by 2015 across each of the UN member countries. To fast track sanitation coverage, the MDGs set up a sanitation target. This target was agreed upon and enlisted as 'Target 7c' to ensure environmental sustainability by aiming to halve the proportion of people without sustainable access to safe drinking water and basic sanitation by 2015. While India did perform well in meeting the water targets, during the MDG era, there was inadequate progress on sanitation. By the end of the MDG period, India had just met its urban sanitation target while its rural sanitation target missed its mark.

With most countries expressing the opinion that setting global development targets was a good idea, another set of targets was agreed upon by the UN in 2015 – the Sustainable Development Goals (SDGs). India has committed to realising the 2030 global agenda in the sanitation sector as per SDG 6 (clean water and sanitation) to 'achieve access to adequate and equitable sanitation and hygiene for all and end open defecation, paying special attention to the needs of women and girls and those in vulnerable situations'. SDGs also emphasise the principle of 'Leave No One Behind' (LNOB) towards achieving goals and targets for all, including the groups being left furthest behind.

Several philanthropic organisations working as international grant-making and implementing agencies have also been active in the sector over the last decade-and-a-half. The largest among them, the Bill and Melinda Gates Foundation (BMGF), has been active in the water sector since 2008. Since 2012, it has increasingly focused its attention on sanitation, and in recent times, it has led to many social innovations in sanitation. Much of BMGF's work in India involves supporting technical and social innovations and sanitation solutions that are cheaper, easier to operate and appropriate in particular contexts. One of its innovative technological exercises has been a global effort to 'Reinvent the Toilet', so that faecal waste can be treated and disposed of right in the toilet to reduce costs of conveyance and centralised treatment.

International partners have played a crucial role in providing the resources (technological and financial) for shaping and implementing various policies, programmes and plans to improve the sanitation situation in India since the 1980s.

## 5. OVERVIEW OF SANITATION POLICIES IN INDIA

Following independence, India adopted a socialist economy, wherein much of the policy direction – even about local affairs – was conceived and financed by the national government. The Planning Commission evolved to be an important stakeholder in the Central Government, and the Five-Year Plans that were developed by the Planning Commission gave direction to development work.

In tracking long-term sanitation policy development in India, the national efforts for financing basic services can be divided into three broad phases. The first phase (1950–1992) began soon after independence and continued till the introduction of the 74th Constitutional Amendment Act, 1992. At the beginning of the first phase, there was a thrust on centrally sponsored schemes for specific cities. The programmes and schemes were entitlement-based, and public services were subsidised to improve access. However, the limited fiscal strength of the Government of India (GOI), and the resulting low-scale funding was not enough to meet the needs of a large and rapidly growing nation. Many pilot projects like the GOI's pilot on urban community development (UCD) and donor-driven pilots, such as the World Bank's sites and service projects, were initiated during this period. The 74th Amendment, in 1992, allowed for the decentralisation and establishment of local governance institutions. This brought a major shift in programme implementation and marked the beginning of the second phase (1992–2005). In 1992, when the GOI was recovering from a financial crisis, an increase in central funding was not viable. There was a large funding deficit in urban infrastructure and basic services. The government assumed the role of a facilitator instead of a provider and worked with CSOs, bilateral and multilateral institutions for making markets work. The first round of public–private partnership (PPP) models was tried out. The focus was on encouraging the debt markets.

This was followed by the final phase (2005 to the present) when the Jawaharlal Nehru National Urban Renewal Scheme (JnNURM) was launched. This scheme involved a large investment in urban infrastructure from the national government; and later in 2014, this period also saw the introduction of the SBM. As part of JnNURM, more than 200 sewerage and wastewater treatment projects were constructed in urban areas at an expenditure of more than Rs 18,000 crore. This phase was marked by fiscal robustness and a shift to reform-based grant funding for core urban infrastructure. It was during this phase that urban sanitation was recognised as key to economic growth and received specific policy attention with the release of the National Urban Sanitation Policy (NUSP) in 2008. NUSP was adopted during the UN International Year of Sanitation (2008). Its goal was articulated as follows:

> All Indian cities and towns should become sanitised, healthy and liveable and ensure and sustain good public health and environmental outcomes for all their citizens with a special focus on hygienic and affordable sanitation facilities for the urban poor and women.

Decentralisation and institutional empowerment at the local body level increased with every phase. Over the years, there has been a significant change in strategy. In the period between the 74th Constitutional Amendment in 1992 and the launch of JnNURM in 2005, entitlement-based, city size and sector-based programmes were implemented. After the introduction of JnNURM in 2005, large grant funding was made available with a shift in focus to large cities. The current urban strategy seeks to delink basic sanitation from reforms. The focus is on demand creation for sanitation and increasing individual responsibility for it. This section discusses the genesis and evolution of India's sanitation policy as reflected in the various FYPs that were adopted since independence.

## *The first phase of the Five-Year Plans*

In 1951, the GOI took the first step towards improving sanitation and health with the launch of the First Five-Year Plan (1951–1956). Health and sanitation were identified as a priority and a budget of Rs 140 crore was sanctioned towards these two necessities. The National Water Supply and Rural Sanitation Programme was launched in 1954 as a part of this plan. It focused on improving water supply in rural areas and was linked to improving sanitary practices. The plan noted that only 43 cities had partial sewerage coverage and that new innovative toilet designs needed to be developed for rural areas (Planning Commission: 1st FYP, n.d.a). By the end of the plan period in 1956, only 100 villages and 32 urban sanitation projects were successful (Planning Commission: 2nd FYP, n.d.b).

The Second Five-Year Plan (1956–1961) allocated more funds to the states and directed them to employ more sanitation workers and engineers to take the sanitation goals further. The Second FYP allocated Rs 53 crore for urban water supply and sanitation, Rs 28 crore for rural water supply and sanitation, and a special grant of Rs 10 crore for urban areas with municipal corporations (Planning Commission: 2nd FYP, n.d.b). By the end of 1961, 1,200 villages had sanitation facilities, an improvement from the results of the First FYP, although still well short of the target (Planning Commission: 3rd FYP, n.d.c).

The Third Five-Year Plan (1961–1966) emphasised the development of agriculture, and the outlay for rural sanitation was reduced to Rs 13 crore – a setback for the minimal sanitation progress India was making. By the end of the 1960s, the phenomenon of urbanisation was beginning to get recognised and the need for expanding basic civic services such as sanitation was now emphasised in almost all policy documents (Planning Commission: 3rd FYP, n.d.c).

The Fourth Five-Year Plan (1969–1974) came amid the need for a dedicated policy paradigm to tackle the challenge of sanitation and acknowledged that it would take time before urban and rural areas could afford full-fledged sewerage and sanitation systems. Technological solutions for sanitation were expected to come from Public Health Engineering Departments. The plan also saw a significant increase in the budgetary allocation towards sanitation, with Rs 407 crore being earmarked for urban sanitation. This exponential increase came in the face of the impetus being placed on inventing new technological solutions to achieve major strides in urban sanitation. Despite the significant focus on the problem of sanitation in the first four FYPs, more than 1 lakh villages and 500 towns were still left without proper water supply and sanitation when the Fifth FYP began.

Environmental acts such as the Water (Prevention and Control) Act, 1974, gained momentum and were enacted to prevent and control water pollution and to restore and maintain the wholesomeness of water (Planning Commission: 4th FYP, n.d.d).

The main thrust of the programmes in the Fifth Five-Year Plan (1974–1979) was directed towards ameliorating the drainage and sanitary conditions of the socially marginalised. This was sought to be achieved by augmenting the programmes for the construction of housing colonies by State Housing Boards. In addition, the construction of sanitary toilets was made a priority, and the FYP made a provision for converting about 30,000–35,000 dry latrines into sanitary latrines covering about 84 towns with sewerage and drainage systems. The newly formed Housing and Urban Development Corporation (HUDCO) and different State Housing Boards were given the responsibility to achieve this target. The Fifth FYP also provided an outlay of Rs 10.27 crore for supporting programmes such as the Public Health Engineering training for about 3,000 personnel and mechanical composting for setting up 27 mechanical compost plants along with 60 mechanical sieve plants in different cities (Planning Commission: 5th FYP, n.d.e).

The Sixth Five-Year Plan (1980–1985) coincided with the beginning of the IDWSSD. This plan also saw the advent of international organisations in the field of sanitation in India, earlier limited to the field of water supply. During this plan period, the UNDP Global Project was initiated in India to assist and promote the installation of water-seal latrines in 110 towns in the seven states of Assam, Bihar, Gujarat, Maharashtra, Rajasthan, Tamil Nadu and Uttar Pradesh. The project aimed at adopting appropriate technologies that would be particularly helpful in smaller towns. In 1980, Integrated Low-Cost Sanitation (ILCS), a centrally sponsored scheme, was launched to convert the existing dry latrines into low-cost, pour-flush latrines and to construct new toilets for economically weaker section (EWS) households without latrines. It aimed to liberate manual scavengers, an imploding and abiding problem that has plagued India over the years. This period also witnessed the evolution of other environmental acts such as the Air (Prevention and Control of Pollution) Act 1981 for the prevention, control and abatement of air pollution and the Environment (Protection) Act 1986 for the protection and improvement of the environment (Planning Commission: 6th FYP, 1981).

The crucial National Master Plan (India) under the International Drinking Water Supply and Sanitation Decade was also brought out in 1983. This comprehensive document was one of the first to talk about soft policies such as community participation, health education in schools and the role of non-governmental organisations (NGOs) in the sphere of Information, Education and Communication (IEC). The foundations for GAP, which was eventually launched in 1985, were also laid down during the Sixth FYP. On the technological front, pilot projects were also taken up in states to find technological solutions for low-cost, water-seal latrines with on-site disposal of human waste.

The advent of the Seventh Five-Year Plan in 1985 fell right in the middle of the Global International Drinking Water Supply and Sanitation Decade, but the sanitation situation in India was still far from ideal. Only 57.27 million people in urban areas, i.e., 33 percent of the urban population had access to sanitation facilities (Census, 1981). The plan also identified the link between low-income levels of the urban poor and low sanitation coverage, reaffirming low-cost sanitation as an important component of India's sanitation improvement. Finally, in 1986, the CRSP was introduced under the National Rural Drinking Water Mission of the Ministry of Rural Development. It was a supply-driven programme based on a subsidy of Rs 2,000 per household to increase rural sanitation coverage. Despite all these measures, the recorded 8 percent improvement in rural sanitation between 1981 and 1991 was way below the target of 25 percent (Planning Commission: 7th FYP, n.d.g.).

HUDCO was asked to finance 50 percent of the cost of the low-cost latrine projects. Additionally, from 1989to 1990, the Urban Low-Cost Sanitation for Liberation of the Scavengers project came under the jurisdiction of the Ministry of Urban Development. Other than the ILCS programme for urban India, much of the focus in this plan as well as future plans hereon was placed on rural sanitation, since the Census (1981) had found that only 1 percent of the rural population had access to safe sanitation. Against a target of covering 25 percent of the rural population by 1990, only 1.82 percent had been achieved (Planning Commission: 7th FYP, n.d.g; National Master Plan – IDWSSD 1981-1990, 1983). Liquid waste management (LWM) had received little direct policy attention till then. In 1985, GAP, which was a centrally funded scheme with external assistance, was launched for pollution abatement and improvement of the water quality of the river Ganga. It sought to prevent pollution and improve the water quality of the Ganga by allocating funds to cities along the river for the construction of STPs. In the first phase, 34 STPs with a capacity of 869 MLD were built, and an additional 18 STPs with a capacity of 129.77 MLD were built in the second phase. In 1995, action plans for other major rivers were merged under the National River Conservation Plan (NRCP). A National River Conservation Directorate was set up under the then Ministry of Environment and Forest (MoEF) to manage the programme. The National Lake Conservation Plan (NLCP) was later initiated to restore urban lakes through an integrated ecosystem approach to protect them from degradation from wastewater discharge.

### The second phase of the Five-Year Plans

The Eighth Five-Year/ Plan (1992–1997), therefore, reinstated the need to address the glaring shortfall in water and sanitation. Emphasis on rural sanitation continued, while efforts in urban areas were refocused on piped drinking water over sanitation. The Ministry of Urban Development formulated an ambitious Accelerated Urban Water Supply (AUWS) pro-gramme that was launched in 1994. About Rs 3,300 crore was allocated for urban sanitation in this plan. The allocation for the ILCS programme was also increased to Rs 550 crore for the Eighth FYP to convert dry latrines into sanitary latrines under the Low-Cost Sanitation Programme (urban) over a period of five years. This was recommended because of the high cost of sewerage and the triple benefit of a low-cost technology option, environ-mental and health benefits and elimination of the dehumanising practice of manual scavenging. The overall assessment of the Eighth FYP showed mixed results. Hardly 13 percent of dry latrines existing from the beginning of the Eighth FYP had been converted into sanitary toilets during the plan period (Planning Commission: 8th FYP, n.d.h).

At the start of the Ninth Five-Year Plan in 1998, 49 percent of the urban population had provision for some sanitary excreta disposal facilities, but only 28 percent had sewerage systems. After the 73rd Constitutional Amendment Act of 1992 was implemented, the role of Panchayati Raj Institutions (PRIs) in rural areas was envisioned to be pivotal to implement a new rural sanitation programme, entitled the Total Sanitation Campaign (TSC). It was CRSP, which was restructured in 1999 as TSC. This new cam-paign aimed to cover toilets in households, *Anganwadis* and schools, mak-ing the district a basic unit. It was based on the principle of Community-Led Total Sanitation (CLTS). It adopted a 'people-centred', 'community-led' and 'demand-driven' approach, where a cash incentive of Rs 1,500 was given by the Central Government and Rs 700 by the state government to households below poverty line (BPL) on the completion of toilet construc-tion. It recognised solid and liquid waste management (SLWM) as a key objective (Planning Commission: 9th FYP, n.d.).

During the initial phases of the Ninth FYP, after the millennium summit of the United Nation in 2000, the MDGs were also adopted for 2000–2015, and for the first time, a need was felt to approach sanitation within a macro frame-work. This framework required an integrated planning approach, which was to work with the help of interdependent infrastructure components, includ-ing water supply, sewerage and sanitation, and waste collection and disposal. In this regard, the Ninth FYP suggested new financial models to overcome the monetary challenges that sanitation systems were faced with. It stated,

> The massive urban growth and the resource constraints would, together, result in a situation where the availability of funds would not keep pace with the growing demand. The urban planners and managers need to be educated and trained to acquire knowledge and skill to change the existing order and help the poor and their settlements.
>
> (Planning Commission: 9th FYP, n.d.i)

The foundations for a programme to recognise individual and community efforts were also discussed in the Ninth FYP, which eventually resulted in the inception of the Nirmal Gram Puraskar (NGP) in 2003. NGP was initiated as an incentive and award programme to achieve ODF status. The national programme awarded *Gram Panchayats* (GPs), blocks and districts for achieving ODF status.

### The third phase of the Five-Year Plans

At the beginning of the 21st century, the population practising OD was pegged at 7.3 million according to the Tenth FYP, and the number of households in need of low-cost sanitation or community toilets was as high as 15 million. The 54th NSS round conducted in 1998 reported that 26 percent of households reported using no latrines, 35 percent reported using septic tanks, and 22 percent reported using a sewerage system (National Sample Survey Organisation – NSSO, 1998). Taking note of this data, the Tenth FYP (2002–2007) noted that as many as 43 percent of households in urban areas had either no latrines or no connection to a septic tank or sewerage (Planning Commission:10th FYP, n.d.j). The total allocation for urban sanitation during this plan period stood at Rs 23,000 crore. Although the policy paradigm on sanitation had recognised the problem of urban sanitation way back in the Second FYP, it began to receive attention only after the 2004 Pune Declaration, followed by the launching of JnNURM in 2005 by the Ministry of Urban Development (MoUD) to improve the provision of basic services for the poor by increasing investment in water and sanitation infrastructure. JnNURM was the single largest initiative ever launched by the GOI to address the problems of urban infrastructure and basic services to the poor with a strong focus on the country's 63 largest cities and towns in a holistic manner. It, however, also dealt with other smaller cities and towns across two broad segments – namely, the sub-mission on Urban Infrastructure and Governance (UIG) for larger cities and the Urban Infrastructure Development Scheme for Small and Medium Towns (UIDSSMT). The GOI's Ministry of Housing and Urban Poverty Alleviation (MoHUPA) was the nodal body for this mission.

The 11th Five-Year Plan (2007–2012) emphasised the need to develop appropriate technology for waste management. The UN's international year of sanitation in 2008 also saw the release of the NUSP. It envisaged all Indian cities and towns becoming sanitised, healthy and liveable, ensuring and sustaining good public health and environmental outcomes for all citizens, with a special focus on the urban poor and women. It recommended the preparation of sanitation strategies for the states and city sanitation plans along the lines of national policy.

The 12th Five-Year Plan (2012–2017) saw TSC being restructured as Nirmal Bharat Abhiyan (NBA) in rural areas. The NBA aimed to achieve *Nirmal Grams* (clean villages) by 2022 through the acceleration of sanitation coverage by enhancing incentives for both BPL and above poverty line (APL) households for the construction of latrines, wherein the national government would award cash incentives of Rs 3,200, the state government would give Rs 1,400 and the beneficiary would pay Rs 900 in cash or labour to subsidise and incentivise some of the costs of latrine construction. It also envisaged the convergence of NBA with the Mahatma Gandhi National Rural Employment Guarantee Scheme (MGNREGS) to enable fund availability for the construction of SLWM facilities, *Anganwadi* toilets and school toilet units in villages. However, the convergence of MGNREGS with NBA created bottlenecks in implantation as funding from different sources created delays, which were again revamped as the national government's flagship mission – Swachh Bharat Mission – targeting both rural and urban sanitation. A key element of this mission was Behaviour Change Communication (BCC) through Community-Led Total Sanitation and the Central Government agreed to provide support of Rs 12,000 for the construction of Individual Household Latrine (IHHL); this payment was to be given to the beneficiary in instalments. Similarly, the 12th FYP underscored improving urban sewerage, drainage and solid waste management services within the overall umbrella scheme of JnNURM-II through structural and governance change at ULB levels and continued capacity augmentation so that these services are provided on a sustained basis. This was to be incentivised through a set of reforms related to urban sanitation, by assisting cities according to their progress in achieving these reforms. Additionally, under JnNURM-II, the NUSP (2008) was envisaged to be effectively implemented so that cities were encouraged to formulate city-wide sanitation plans, while the states adopted State Sanitation Strategies (Planning Commission: 12th FYP, n.d.k).

In October 2014, SBM (Urban) was launched by the Ministry of Housing and Urban Affairs (MoHUA) to eliminate the practice of OD, ensure municipal solid waste management, and eradicate manual scavenging. The present national government's push for sanitation is evident from its mission mode to build toilets, but building the superstructure is not enough to address the sanitation challenge of India. Another major highlight of the 12th FYP was a shift from MDGs to SDGs in 2015. Goal 6 of the SDGs currently being formulated for 2015–2030 recognises water and sanitation as distinct goals. This also corresponds with the launch of AMRUT and the Smart City Mission (SCM) in 2015, which aims at transforming urban India. The AMRUT and SCM both prioritised urban sanitation, thereby recognising that improper access to basic civic services like safe drinking water and improved sanitation is intrinsically connected to underdevelopment, poverty, gender oppression, environment and human health. It also accepted that access to improved sanitation is imperative for good health and safe drinking water supply and that access to functional toilet facilities, reducing the practice of OD and adopting positive hygiene behaviour significantly reduce morbidity, mortality and stunting among children.

AMRUT allowed for septage management investments for urban areas, which encouraged states to submit plans for safe and sustainable faecal sludge management solutions. Further, the publishing of the National Policy on Faecal Sludge and Septage Management (FSSM) (2017) and FSSM operative guidelines as well as the state policies of 19 states and Union Territories (2018) helped scale up approaches to safely managed sanitation, especially for urban India. From just one Faecal Sludge Treatment Plant (FSTP) in 2014, there are more than 120 FSTPs in operation today; and according to some estimates, 550 FSTPs are under consideration and construction. India has witnessed a significant leap in five years to tackle issues of OD and adopt faecal sludge management (FSM).

Despite the FYP process and the former Planning Commission that oversaw it, being recast, the GOI announced a renewal of its focus on water and sanitation in 2019 and created the Jal Shakti Ministry at the national level. The Jal Shakti Ministry has brought together the functions of the former ministries of Water Resources and that of Drinking Water and Sanitation under one umbrella. The government's view is that this will allow for smoother coordination between the policies and programmes related to the various issues of water. As shared by experts, 'If 2014-19 was the phase to drive and upscale sanitation in the country, then 2019-24 will drop the spotlight on water' (Down to Earth, 2019). In the face of an ever-increasing water crisis, the need for ensuring a sound infrastructure for piped water facilities, especially in local areas, will require strong political as well as policy commitment from all stakeholders. Earlier, the GOI had launched the Jal Shakti Abhiyan and the Jal Jeevan Mission under the Jal Shakti Ministry to underscore the relevance of interlinking water with the ongoing sanitation programme. The Jal Jeevan Mission (JJM) aims to ensure piped water supply to all rural households by 2024. This special thrust on water accentuates the need to align focus from just sanitation to integrated water and sanitation, including water supply augmentation, demand management and recycling of wastewater and FSM as the sustainable solution, going forward. The JJM provides an opportunity to view water and wastewater in a circular manner and develop integrated solutions in urban and rural areas. This new government programme aims to adopt subsidiarity as a key principle. This concept is being expressed as the ownership and management of assets and services at the lowest level of decision-making, i.e., decisions made by the stakeholders most affected by the asset or facility. This is important to achieve the goal of sustainable sanitation.

## 6. INNOVATIONS FOR MEETING UNMET SOCIAL NEEDS OF IMPROVED SANITATION

Drawing on the evolution of India's sanitation policy, this chapter demonstrates how sanitation policies in the past have evolved through a process of social innovation. Such innovative approaches can play a significant role in contributing to India's aspiration to meet the global agenda delineated by SDG 6 on clean water and sanitation.

Illustrating the urban sanitation journey, this chapter critically reflects upon the challenges in this sector. These include building capacities of all stakeholders; sustained access and functionality of the sanitation infrastructure; safe and scientific solid waste, faecal sludge and septage management; complete prohibition of manual scavenging and reaching the most marginalised.

Many social innovations that the CSOs piloted and helped scale are now well embedded in public programmes executed by governments in the sanitation sector. Thus, the policies evolved across the FYPs since independence has benefited from social innovations pioneered by the CSOs. In light of the steadily evolving challenges in the Indian sanitation situation, a framework that allows us to recognise the contributions of CSOs and the social innovations that they have been instrumental in pioneering can provide an invaluable understanding of ways to move beyond conventional solutions to meet unmet needs. This framework should be robust enough to catalyse the various changes – social, cultural and technological – that various state policies and development partners seek to make. The subsequent chapters in this book discuss and analyse some of the most important CSO-crafted social innovations that have now become a mainstream part of public policy in India.

Technological innovation in safe toilet design for India has been a critical innovation that has allowed for the penetration of toilets in both cities and villages. These innovations have had to respond to cultural, climatic, limited in-house piped water availability and economic contexts that are different from developed countries where toilets came to be in universal use much earlier. The technologies that were developed in the early phase – from the 1950s till the early 1970s – are still in use today, incrementally evolving and improving. Pour-flush, single pit toilets, the development of the ventilated improved pit (VIP) and the twin pit ventilated latrine are the most significant technologies developed and implemented at scale by these institutions in India. Since the ILCS in urban areas during the Sixth FYP and the TSC in the 1990s, the twin pit ventilated, pour-flush latrine has become the technology of choice for rural sanitation as well as in small-town India. This technological innovation, building on the work of the CSOs, has had a far-reaching impact on improving the sanitation situation in the country.

Therefore, ever since the early phase of sanitation policy and programmes supported by governments in India, CSOs have supported the pursuit of improving the sanitation situation. More recently too, as discussed extensively in the following chapters, with the emphasis on public policy moving from basic sanitation to environmental sanitation, the development of technologies for faecal sludge management and decentralised wastewater treatment pioneered by CSOs are today rapidly spreading across smaller cities in the country, funded through national and state government programmes.

CSOs have also contributed to social innovations in sanitation by developing service delivery institutional models for sanitation operations. The operational model for pay-and-use community toilets demonstrated that users are willing to pay for clean and hygienic sanitation services. The recent innovations around models for city-wide faecal sludge management systems are now well-established models across cities for environmental sanitation.

The CSOs have also pioneered the capacity development of public institutions to scale up social innovations. Public institutions such as water and sanitation parastatal bodies, state and national ministries and departments as well as environmental protection agencies have been capacitated by the CSOs in many geographies with support from international agencies. Governments have been increasingly relying on CSOs and technical agencies for training staff within government programmes as centres of excellence. CSOs have also played strong advocacy roles in enacting and ensuring the implementation of sanitation laws and regulations, including the issues of manual scavenging. Further to faecal sludge management, several CSOs have assisted governments in developing and implementing sanitation regulations.

The need for Behaviour Change Communication has been realised as critical, as many toilets that were constructed under various programmes were not effectively used by the community due to prevalent cultural practices. While mainly used in rural areas, given its higher utility in these regions, the innovation of the Community-Led Sanitation Model has now become central to national policies and programmes. Other tools for behaviour change, including communication campaigns and the sanitation marketing model, are also being extensively used in present-day sanitation programmes across rural and urban India.

# 2 Social Innovation in Urban Sanitation
## Experiences from India

## 1. INTRODUCTION

This chapter examines the literature on social innovations from the 1990s onwards and applies the conceptual frameworks from this to gain a deeper understanding of the changes being made in the context of Indian urban sanitation. In doing so, it draws extensively on specific examples positioned from all parts of the country where experiments and interventions have been made in urban sanitation and have placed households and communities at the heart of such changes.

It begins with arriving at a working definition of the term social innovation and then delves into different components of these innovations in the context of urban sanitation in India. To do this, it examines community-based innovations in urban sanitation undertaken by a host of civil society organisations (CSOs) like the Centre for Policy Research (CPR), Centre for Science and Environment (CSE), Centre for Urban and Regional Excellence (CURE), Consortium for DEWATS Dissemination (CDD), Development Alternatives (DA), Gramalaya, Nidan, Participatory Research in Asia (PRIA), Safai Karmachari Andolan (SKA) and Urban Management Centre (UMC). The social innovations in urban sanitation undertaken by these organisations are not about using technology alone – though technological changes are part of many of these initiatives – but equally about methodologies to involve people and local communities in generating solutions to the urban sanitation situation in India, as described in the previous chapter.

The case studies indicate four key features of social innovations in urban sanitation – the fact that these represent a coming together of existing elements rather than representing new inventions per se; that almost all of them cut across organisational, sectoral and disciplinary boundaries; that they set in motion a set of new relationships between previously disjointed individuals and groups, thereby carrying the potential to trigger off innovations; and that they generate behaviour changes that are sometimes more noticeable and at other times more subtle. These characteristics of hybridity, intersectionality, relationship building (Mulgan et al., 2007) and behaviour

DOI: 10.4324/9781003197102-2

change present the possibility that these experiments in social innovations in urban sanitation can be scaled up. The chapter concludes by examining some of the challenges involved in this critical process of scaling up, which is needed to create the necessary social impact in the arena of urban sanitation.

We observe that while the practice of social innovations may be abundant, a systematic inquiry into various aspects of economic and social development, using this lens, is not common, particularly in the Global South. Taking a cue from this, we examine the specific arena of urban sanitation in India to try and uncover approaches to sanitation challenges that have been around us over the years but failed to receive attention in terms of their innovative potential and ability to drive social change that is of direct benefit to vulnerable social segments.

We begin by arriving at a working definition of the term 'social innovation' and then delve into different aspects of these innovations in urban sanitation in India, drawing from the field-based research and case studies documented. We conclude with some pointers on the impact of such social innovations and the challenges faced in scaling them up – a theme we will revisit in greater detail in the concluding chapter of this book.

## 2. SOCIAL INNOVATION: WHAT DOES IT MEAN?

The notion of social innovation is often presented as a bundle of meanings with loosely defined boundaries. Though the term 'innovation' was typically associated with technology that drives economic development (McNeill, 2012), social innovation as an idea dates back to the beginning of the 19th century when it entered the vocabulary in the aftermath of the French Revolution. Godin (2012) focuses on the developments in the innovations discourse post-1830s and presents a genealogy of 'social' innovation by moving away from a purely technological understanding of the concept. Countering the perception that social innovation is a new concept, as represented in academic works of scholars like Drucker (1986), Mulgan (2006) and Godin (2012), points out that even 'the social reformer is/was a social innovator' and that anything new in 'social' matters could be called social innovation.

The concept of social innovation that originated in the 1950s coincided with a phase when state interventions were increasingly linking social problems with technological solutions. In that context, social innovation emerged as a response to this continued hegemony of technological innovation (ibid.). Deepening this approach, Drucker (1986) forwards the hypothesis that innovation is an economic or social term rather than a technical term alone and points to the danger of over-dependence on science and technology as a driver of social change (Drucker, 1986). The vocabulary on technology became that of technological innovation, and sociologists resurrected the term social innovation.

Societies develop and transform because of innovation and in turn influence the innovation (Lapierre, 1968). Social innovation includes any type of innovation in the realm of political or organisational innovation as long as it has some 'social' orientation. It is also more or less what is largely known as social policy and reform. Social innovation privileges the non-institutional, the 'alternative' and the 'marginal'. It is an innovation of a public or collaborative nature. Barroso (2011) has emphasised social innovation as meeting unmet social needs and improving social outcomes. It taps creativity to find new ways of meeting pressing social needs, which are not adequately met by the market or the public sector and are directed towards vulnerable social groups.

Zapf (1991) discusses social innovation in the context of modernisation theory, defining it as 'a new way of doing things, especially new organizational devices, new regulations, new living arrangements, that change the direction of social change, attain goals better than old practices, become institutionalized and prove to be worth imitating'. We also note with Mulgan et al. (2007) that unlike business innovation, which is driven by profit maximisation, social innovations are motivated by a concern of meeting a social need and are diffused through organisations whose primary purposes are social development. Social innovation is, above all, democratic, citizen- or community-oriented and user-friendly; it assigns significance to what is personalised, small, holistic and sustainable; its methods are diverse, not restricted to standard science and include open innovation, user participation, cafés, ethnography, action research, etc. (Murray et al., 2010).

Essaying a similar strain of thought, Cajaiba-Santana (2014) posits that the intentionality of social innovation is what sets it apart from technical innovation. Unlike purely technical innovation, which is often achieved by assembling past technical discoveries to solve a particular technical problem, social innovation brings up social change that cannot be built up based on established practices and, therefore, is a clear break from the existing social context and norms. Since social innovation centres on the process of social change itself, it is a broader process than social entrepreneurship (Cunha et al., 2015). It envisages a potential reality and brings together resources that can make it happen (ibid.). Disagreeing that social innovation is merely a buzzword in academics, Pol and Ville (2009) lay down a pragmatic definition – 'an innovation is termed a social innovation if the implied new idea has the potential to improve either the quality or quantity of life'. They highlight the need to institutionalise social innovation through incentives because, as Mulgan (2006) points out, social innovations may take decades to create an impact on the ground. He reminds us that to transit from a promising pilot idea to becoming a mainstream product, it is necessary to tap into networks between those working on the ground and those in policymaking circles.

## 3. SOCIAL INNOVATION AS NEW IDEAS TO MEET UNMET NEEDS

The deficits in urban sanitation in India indicate that the challenge of sanitation in the country is of such magnitude that it has held up international progress in this arena. The case studies on urban sanitation curated and analysed from different parts of the country indicate that in response to this situation and even before the launch of the much-publicised, central flagship mission of 2014 – Swachh Bharat Mission (SBM) – there were several innovations in urban sanitation. These had, however, not received sufficient attention in the absence of a major thrust and framework with the explicit aim of addressing the challenge of urban sanitation.

The basic notion of social innovation hinges on new ideas that meet unmet needs (Barroso, 2011). The case studies on urban sanitation projects that we have used in this book throw up a variety of approaches and ideas on how to engage with the challenge of urban sanitation in India. Some of these ideas are:

A. The basic intertwining of sanitation with a much wider 'participatory, efficient and sustainable water management paradigm' is integral to any social innovation in urban sanitation. The innovative idea here is to **include wastewater treatment or management and faecal sludge management within the sanitation issue and link it to the overall issues of environmental pollution**. A conscious attempt in this direction was made by the CSE. At the core of this social innovation was the response to an old problem of neglecting onsite waste management like septic tanks and linking it with the larger sanitation issue.

B. A second innovation in urban sanitation was to **encourage a home-based solution to people's needs for toilets and taps through a participatory process and by placing users at the heart of the process**. The innovative idea led by CURE rests on the belief that people, including the poor, have local wisdom, can self-organise as networks, overcome personal differences and collaborate in reshaping their environments.

C. A third socially innovative idea was to **improvise ideas field tested from rural sanitation** such as the construction of leach pit toilets, eco-san toilets made with septic tanks and community toilets **for the urban context by placing behaviour change at the core of the innovation** rather than merely physical construction of toilets. Such an initiative was led by Gramalaya. The behaviour change relied on changing mindsets by providing opportunities for marginalised communities to work together on a common theme, place women in decision-making roles and emphasise values of self-reliance at sites around individual households and schools, which provided the primary sites of intervention in the urban context.

D. Another social innovation initiated by Nidan in urban sanitation came from the idea that **hawkers and vendors** could be **at the forefront of** sanitation issues in the urban context by recognising it as their human right and providing slum communities access to toilets along with advocacy work regarding toilet usage.

E. **Placing the neglected issue of manual scavenging at the heart of the sanitation issue** formed the bedrock of another social innovation, which then emerged into a movement to abolish the dehumanising practice of manual scavenging and promote dignified rehabilitation for those who have taken up this work. *The evolution of the SKA into a people's movement based on the values of dignity, self-respect and equality is itself the story of social innovation at work.*

F. Another social innovation in urban sanitation led by UMC is based on **providing a chain of deliverables in the sanitation sector that works towards professionalising and innovating urban management** by making organisational interventions as a 'friend of the city' and acknowledging that change can occur only when local governments take on sanitation as part of the larger process of municipal development.

G. Starting **sanitation work with green technology materials and capacity building of masons** to build toilets have been at the kernel of yet another social innovation, which emphasises behaviour change communication by using the youth as agents of change to identify and articulate urban issues, propose solutions and take actions for the future. This approach has been followed by Development Alternatives.

H. An innovation in urban sanitation, **Decentralised Wastewater Treatment Systems (DEWATS), specifically focuses on eco-friendly, low-maintenance technology suitable for managing a wide range of wastewater at reasonable costs.** Since this is a technological innovation, it focuses on providing facilities to train, design and apply research and development along with knowledge management. It does this by targeting low-income communities.

At the heart of many of these social innovations in urban sanitation lies the idea of behaviour change, which is facilitated at times through a conscious process of strategic communication but can also happen more organically at other times through a process of co-learning between government agencies, the social sector and local communities.

In subsequent chapters, this book will describe how, over the years, social innovations adapted existing technologies to 'meet unmet needs' by introducing green technology to decentralised wastewater management or encouraging home-based solutions to people's needs for toilets through improvised ideas field tested in rural sanitation for urban use (such as the construction of leach pit toilets). It will draw attention to strategies, methods and tools to organise the unorganised communities for amplifying their voices to access urban sanitation services as well as realising rights and dignity. It will highlight how an organisation created a movement to abolish manual scavenging, making the restoration of dignity, safety and health the core of their social innovation on urban sanitation. The book will also touch upon social innovations such as providing a chain of deliverables in the sanitation sector and organising hawkers and vendors to be at the forefront of urban sanitation issues. Finally, it will examine how strategic communication can play a role in behaviour change when a socially innovative initiative is started in urban sanitation.

## 4. CHARACTERISTICS OF SOCIAL INNOVATIONS IN THE URBAN SANITATION SECTOR IN INDIA

In light of the above discussion – and drawing on the work by Mulgan et al. (2007) – we look at four characteristics of social innovations in the urban sanitation sector in India: (i) hybridity, (ii) intersectionality, (iii) relationship building and (iv) behaviour change. In this connection, we examine examples drawn from various case studies as part of the urban sanitation project, which are described in detail in other parts of this book.

### Hybridity

Usually, social innovations involve hybrids of existing elements rather than being wholly new in themselves (Mulgan et al., 2007). Several experiences from urban sanitation indicate such a hybrid approach. In the examples gathered from the field, instances of such hybridity were apparent in socially innovative approaches to urban sanitation in the work of several CSOs like CSE, CURE, UMC and DA.

The Decentralised Waste Water Treatment (DWWT) system in urban sanitation promoted and implemented by CSE, for instance, has used soil biotechnology and green technology for water purification using a natural, high-efficiency oxidation process that combines sedimentation, infiltration and biodegradation processes. The system also consists of coarse or fine screen chambers, or grit chambers, for preliminary treatment, treated water tanks, piping, pumps and electrical and civil works. In all of this, it brings together diverse elements such as capacity-building initiatives on citywide sanitation for urban local bodies (ULBs) located along the Ganga basin, the strengthening capacities of city officials in preparing city sanitation plans and septage management projects, decentralised wastewater treatment programme and shit flow diagram within its overall paradigm of promoting sustainable and equitable development.

Another example of how diverse elements are brought together in social innovations in urban sanitation is afforded by the work of CURE, which has designed the cluster septic tank (CST) to counter the problems of unusable community toilets, badly designed private septic tanks that run the risk of creating sink holes and the overall issue of open defecation, which is not only unhygienic but dangerous, especially for women and children. The CST has proved to be a low-cost solution installed in partnership with people and has offered a new template for in-house sanitation services in unplanned urban fringes, bringing sanitation to even the poorest of households. In implementing its work, CURE has embraced a hybrid approach in so far as it combines new technological ideas generated by its in-house expertise with community-based solutions and resources to co-design and co-implement interventions.

The work of UMC, which works with ULBs to support improvements in data reliability as well as service delivery, is based on providing a chain of deliverables in the urban sanitation sector by bringing together multiple elements such as collecting information from the ground, conducting situation assessment through performance monitoring, advocating best practices through their city links initiative, formulating city sanitation plans, auditing existing facilities and suggesting improvisation in procedures and systems of the sector along with infrastructural improvements.

Another example of the hybrid approach to social innovation in urban sanitation can be seen in the work of DA, which started urban sanitation work in the last decade with a small initiative to build the capacities of masons to construct toilets and facilitate technological innovations related to pre-fabricated toilets with recyclable materials. In developing capacities of masons, DA brought multiple distinct elements such as technologically innovative toilet solutions and behaviour change communication with the latter being led by social media initiatives spearheaded by the youth. Systematic assessment of environmental quality, including sanitation of major cities, awareness led by school children to influence communities, action demonstrating good practices and finally advocacy for informed policy change form part of the '4 As' approach – focusing on attractions (natural and artificial), actors (hosts and tourists), actions and atmosphere – that represents a hybrid approach to urban sanitation.

## Intersectionality

As Mulgan (2006) points out social innovations have to invariably cross the 'chasm' – from being promising pilot ideas to becoming mainstream products – and in this process fully tap into the role of a network of CSOs working on the ground and in policy-making circles. The case studies that we have drawn upon in this book demonstrate that social and technological innovations are predominantly diffused across organisational, sectoral, and disciplinary boundaries through CSOs that are primarily motivated by the goal of meeting a social need and creating an impact on the ground. This intersectionality is a key feature of social innovations as they require finances, authority and ideas to come together.

A research and advocacy organisation like CSE, for instance, receives funding from the Government of India's (GOI's) Ministry of Housing and Urban Affairs (MoHUA) and the Ministry of Environment, Forests, and Climate Change (MoEFCC) and works with the state governments as well as the erstwhile Planning Commission. CSE has operated across boundaries and diffused its ideas through its Centre for Excellence on Sustainable Water Management, imparting its knowledge and skills on rainwater harvesting and faecal sludge management to urban sanitation stakeholders, including government officials across various states, training trainers as well as researchers working in the area of sustainable development. Similarly, CURE has brought together its in-house experts – such as planners, engineers and architects – and members of the community, particularly the urban poor, to co-design and co-implement interventions on sanitation. Its intersectoral outreach includes experts in information technology (IT) so that smart IT-based solutions can be used for city sanitation planning. We see the same kind of intersectoral cross-cutting in the work of Gramalaya, which advocates a low-cost toilet model known as eco-san toilets that are affordable and acceptable by the local communities of India's coastal and delta regions. These toilets are constructed above the ground level with the wash water being diverted to the kitchen gardens and prevented from mingling with human faeces. While carrying out this work, Gramalaya interfaces with the government, households and schools, which were the primary sites of intervention along with CSOs, such as the HT Parekh Foundation.

Nidan, which works on sanitation issues, offers an example of the conscious use of policy advocacy in urban sanitation regarding toilet use and hardware development. To influence policy, and implement process and behaviour change, Nidan has initiated several policy-level dialogues while leveraging its relationships with worker groups from informal settlements. Nidan's work has brought together government agencies, networks, slum communities, schools and *Anganwadis*, and sanitation service providers in a deliberately crafted multisectoral approach that works to break through various development silos and make sanitation a citywide agenda. As part of this intersectoral approach, it has developed the idea of 'sanitation marts', which would address the livelihood opportunities of the urban poor who can become contractors and masons.

We also draw on the example of the SKA, which has been mobilising sanitation workers against the dehumanising occupation of scavenging and asking for dignified rehabilitation for those who have undertaken the work of physically removing untreated human excreta. SKA invested substantially in building awareness of the equality and dignity of every human being, directly confronting issues related to caste and patriarchy. It envisions that eradicating manual scavenging will break the link imposed by the caste system between birth and dehumanising occupations. In carrying out this work, it has worked in partnership with other CSOs committed to the rights of scheduled castes and other marginalised communities and *safai karmachari* such as the All India Sweepers Community, the Adar Shila, the Valmiki Samaj, Solidarity Group for Children against discrimination and exclusion across India's states and Union Territories of Bihar, Delhi, Gujarat, Haryana, Jammu and Kashmir, Madhya Pradesh, Punjab,

Tamil Nadu, Uttar Pradesh and West Bengal. Taking the idea of dignity and rehabilitation of those working on the issues of manual scavenging also means engaging with the media and working with district and administrative authorities.

Another social innovation in urban sanitation that brings together universities, governments and technocrats is the work of UMC, which provides a chain of deliverables in the sanitation sector. It works towards professionalising and innovating urban management by making organisational interventions a 'friend of the city' and acknowledging that change can occur only when local governments take on sanitation as part of the larger process of municipal development. UMC works with a few ULBs to support improvements in data reliability as well as actual service delivery in septage management in nonsewered cities, low-cost wastewater treatment methods, public grievance redressal systems, and management information systems for improved reliability of data and drinking water surveillance procedures for ULBs. UMC has been a pioneer in training and capacity building of city managers and has also been the back office now for online courses on SBM for city managers. It is currently handling the end-to-end development of 85 tutorials, including content development, moderation and a digital resource library. Given the nature of its work, UMC's interventions in urban sanitation involved bringing together the practitioner and the academic through the Habitat Management Course at the Centre for Environmental Planning and Technology (CEPT) University, Ahmedabad, engaging with the city, central and state governments for various urban management aspects, bringing in technocrats for data mapping, visualisation and analysis while promoting appropriate technological platforms and advocating through innovative media and communication tools such as films, theatres, books and blogs.

DA has worked with an array of stakeholders – community members, multilateral donor agencies, policymakers at different tiers of government, private sector representatives and CSOs – to influence the policies and practices on sustainable development, including sustainable sanitation. Similarly, CDD works on urban sanitation, environment and water security for the disadvantaged poor with decentralisation and community participation as its key approach. It has worked with a network of more than 20 like-minded partner organisations across the country, which consist of different government agencies, not-for-profit entities, educational institutions and private service providers.

### Relationship building

Due to the intersectionality across different disciplines and sectors in almost all social innovations studied in this research, a set of new relationships between previously disjointed individuals and groups has resulted in a diffusion of ideas, where each idea has the potential to trigger innovations. The role of the state and government-funded programmes is often seen to provide spaces for forming new relationships. In sanitation, in particular, earlier state programmes like the Central Rural Sanitation Programme (1986) and National Drinking Water Mission (1986) are examples that allowed multiple CSOs and individuals in technological and social innovations to work together to scale new models for sanitation and embed change in social norms.

PRIA's work with informal settlements has transcended interventions with the urban poor to include middle-income residents, professionals, traders, market associations, local media and academic institutions, facilitating them to work with ULBs in a citywide, inclusive sanitation framework. The collaborative effort of CPR, practical action and CDD demonstrates low-cost, decentralised, inclusive and sustainable sanitation service delivery solutions. Such a collaborative partnership furthered efforts in improving sanitation access for all households and integrating faecal sludge management into the sanitation value chain by enabling institutional and financial arrangements and increased private sector participation.

In the global context, India has remained the site where sanitation conditions are among the weakest. Within this context, earlier national flagships programmes like the Central Rural Sanitation Programme (CRSP) and Total Sanitation Campaign (TSC) and the current SBM and Atal Mission for Rejuvenation and Urban Transformation (AMRUT) have provided a platform for CSOs with different approaches but working for a similar theme to further the critical issues of meeting unmet needs in urban sanitation. Knowledge-based advocacy efforts from national and international CSO networks like Freshwater Action Network (FANSA), South Asia Conference on Sanitation (SACOSAN), International Water Association (IWA) and National Faecal Sludge and Septage Management (NFSSM) Alliance are some of the groups who have helped to build consensus and drive the discourse on specific issues of urban sanitation.

## Behaviour change

Integral to the process of social innovation is the behaviour change of all stakeholders as they interact and engage in a mutual process of co-learning. The parties carrying out the social innovation, the policymakers and the targeted 'beneficiaries' within the community undergo changes that sometimes occur more noticeably and sometimes in a more subtle way. Behaviour change is sometimes actively facilitated by a process of strategic communication, which involves applying the processes, strategies and principles of communication to reach out to people to influence attitudes and bring about positive social change. The case studies have indicated several such instances when social innovation in urban sanitation tried to consciously bring about this change of attitude and behaviour either through campaign messaging or the use of mass media and interpersonal messages directed at the urban poor. The behaviour change in urban sanitation is aimed not just at encouraging the community to construct and use toilets but to embrace the complete sanitation value. It is also directed at government agencies to encourage thinking across developmental silos and acknowledge that urban sanitation is not just an issue for the municipality or urban ministry but also linked closely to health, social work, education and livelihoods.

## 5. THE WAY FORWARD

Despite the achievements in the sanitation sector following large policy pushes exemplified by SBM and AMRUT, the key challenge lies in whether these interventions have significantly impacted the lives of marginalised communities and those of women. Hazardous cleaning of septic tanks, the unabated practice of manual scavenging and the increasing incidents of deaths of manual scavengers have brought issues of dignity and safety of workers to the national agenda. Additionally, issues about proper containment, transportation, disposal, recycling and re-use of faecal waste are yet to be fully addressed. This is where the role of social innovation comes in – new ideas to meet unmet social needs – related in this case to the enormous challenge of providing an urban sanitation infrastructure to the growing population of India's cities.

The latter part of the decade has seen an addition of a significant number of toilets but without a commensurate spread of the sewer network. As a result, most of these newly constructed toilets are connected to onsite sanitation systems across rural and urban areas. Such onsite systems, if constructed wisely, can enable a safe containment and treatment of waste. It is this thrust on non-networked onsite systems that has led to various states coming up with their urban sanitation policies with a special emphasis on developing decentralised facilities for faecal sludge management, and this has created spaces for social innovations that could be of direct benefit to marginalised communities.

Social innovation in urban sanitation has had important social consequences by 'organising the unorganised', 'servicing the voices of the poor' and 'ensuring a comprehensive dialogue between different stakeholders'. This idea of inclusive sanitation is exemplified in the concept of citywide inclusive sanitation (Schrecongost, 2020), which links all benefits from adequate sanitation service delivery outcomes. Human waste is safely managed along the whole sanitation service chain; effective resource recovery and re-use are considered; a diversity of technical solutions is embraced for adaptive, mixed and incremental approaches; and onsite as well as sewerage solutions are combined in either centralised or decentralised systems to better respond to the realities of cities in developing countries. The spirit of citywide inclusive sanitation assumes that the consequences of inadequate sanitation affect everyone, as human waste and its pathogens recognise no boundaries and spread freely across urban areas. This is why city leaders, as well as individuals, need to use their political capital and power to drive a coherent citywide strategy that delivers on sanitation as a human right. With 'business as usual' not working anymore, only a radical shift in mindsets and practices, with sustained behaviour change, will make a difference. This radical shift would invariably require the engagement of all stakeholders – formal and informal – and political accountability of all citizens, rich and poor alike, with enhanced attention to the needs of the poor and vulnerable in urban sanitation. Such an initiative would require collaboration between many actors, including the national, sub-national and city/municipal governments; utilities and municipal service providers; business and the private sector; civil society, local and international non-governmental organisations (NGOs); bilateral and multilateral donors, and private foundations; as well as academia and, importantly, communities themselves. Effecting this combination mandates a paradigm shift in the way in which urban sanitation is perceived in the country. This is exactly where the importance of social innovation can be underscored with its key feature of building linkages and collaborations across multiple fault lines and boundaries.

At the same time, it is important to emphasise that the idea of social innovation in urban sanitation needs to go further than its traditional role of facilitating a social impact of technology that is already available. There is a need to integrate innovations across the entire value chain within urban sanitation. This would involve not just a diffusion of pro-poor innovations but also a whole range of other initiatives such as mobilisation of the poor, advocating for better liaison with the system, creating both demand and supply for sanitation services and building local capabilities when it comes to sanitation networks. This is possible if a National System of Innovation (NSI) framework is adopted for urban sanitation. As suggested by Ramani et al. (2017), NSI offers a system where the creation, commercialisation and adoption of innovations are collective processes embedded within a system specific to the country concerned. This means that the country's social innovation must be driven by local issues and shaped by the contours of its local cultural and socio-economic realities.

For meaningful social innovations to animate the arena of urban sanitation, it has to move towards a holistic idea of what constitutes innovation and who can initiate it. Traditional schools of thought would consider social innovation to be outside the purview of the state's ambit as it is doing what the governments could not do. However, the time has come to abandon such compartmentalised imaginations on social innovation. There is a need for the state, civil society and business communities to come together and complement each other's efforts to build an NSI that is specific to urban sanitation.

Looking at the innovations in urban sanitation, we are left asking how do we make innovations 'pro-poor' when enterprises that drive some of these innovations are 'for-profit'? How can the idea of coming up with pro-poor innovations be sustained if innovations are marketed to people at a profit, turning them into consumers? Can social innovation be sustained and encouraged without allowing individuals who pioneer these innovations to earn profit?

This is where the role of governments (both national and state) becomes prominent. By making way for social innovations in their stated policies and programmes, governments can facilitate new technology creation and business entrepreneurship in the sanitation sector. What is also important is that such policies emphasise sufficiently recognising the contribution of small organisations to social innovation. While organisations like Gramalaya and Sulabh International do serve as examples of successful models of social entrepreneurship in sanitation, they continue to be exceptions and not a product of the ecosystem. The onus of creating and sustaining such an ecosystem lies with the government. While the model of social entrepreneurship has survived and thrived in other countries (such as the USA, for instance) independent of the government, expecting it to be replicated in India would not be prudent. This is because urban sanitation remains an important and unfulfilled promise made by the welfare state to its people. Just as decentralised sanitation systems have come to replace large sewerage systems as the major thrust for sanitation infrastructure, the social entrepreneurship model requires a push from the state to become one of the primary anchors for effecting social innovation. There is a limit to what individuals can achieve in terms of innovating with technologies, organising the poor or advocating for the safety and dignity of the workers. Such initiatives have to be recognised and incentivised by bringing a model where entrepreneurs can come together to invest capital and other resources to innovate (not just technologically but also culturally and socially), thereby giving shape to one of the first NSI in the field of urban sanitation that can be subsequently emulated by other sectors, such as education and healthcare.

This book touches upon various facets of social innovation that have impacted the urban sanitation landscape of India. Our ground studies have indicated that mere attention to infrastructural needs is not enough, and they have to be related to social and cultural realities that pervade notions around sanitation in India. Efforts towards building collaborations and partnerships, engagement with social sector organisations, community-based organisations, citizens, media and the private sector, are key to sustaining the innovations that have taken place to date. Sustaining these innovations will be contingent upon the successful decentralisation vis-à-vis planning, installation, ownership, operation and maintenance on the part of the state, on the one hand, and successful mobilisation vis-à-vis advocacy, organisation building, awareness and capability enhancement on the part of CSOs and social entrepreneurs, on the other.

# 3 Organisation Building for Inclusive Urban Sanitation

## Organising the Unorganised

## 1. INTRODUCTION

Building collectives of the poor and marginalised in urban settings has evolved as a powerful strategy for accessing basic urban services, including sanitation by underserved communities. Collectivisation is at the core of any strategy where communities, earlier perceived as voiceless, demand and receive improved public services. These communities themselves often seek the support of other civil society organisations and mobilise their members in identifying problems, strategising actions and finding out solutions by partnering with local authorities.

This chapter focuses on the organisation building of the poor and marginalised to meet their unmet sanitation needs and bring about social transformation by mobilising the collective voices of people in ways that they become part of the solutions. Organising groups and collectives, developing communication channels between privileged and underprivileged urban residents, creating participatory and democratic forums and facilitating dialogues between underprivileged communities and local authorities are key elements in this strategy. Sanitation in its materiality, and when seen as a chain of associated activities, is both a private good in some parts and a public good in most others. The public good implies that for it to be successfully provided and accessed as per established standards, it needs to benefit the whole community, leaving no one behind. As sanitation infrastructure and services become more available to people at large, to ensure that no one is left behind, organisation building of the poor and marginalised has emerged as a crucial component for increasing access to safely managed systems for the community to create positive impacts on public health and the environment.

The necessity to connect these collectives of underserved marginalised people with other stakeholders, such as the government and civil society, the communities also need to foster intersectionality in their organisation to emerge as a successful social innovation.

The chapter illustrates and analyses different approaches by examining specific cases of organisation building in marginalised and underserved

DOI: 10.4324/9781003197102-3

communities to bring changes in their quality of life by improving access to services, ensuring safety and justice and making governance institutions more accountable and transparent.

## 2. COLLECTIVISATION AND ORGANISATION BUILDING AS SOCIAL INNOVATION

An integral part of any social innovation approach that aims to improve access to the marginalised and underserved involves amplifying their voices by collectivising their strengths to make them and the challenges they face visible to policymakers. Positive actions in support of the marginalised would invariably require bringing inclusiveness in various government processes at various levels to identify and define issues, develop insights into the issues through the collection and collective interpretation of data, planning, assessing the solutions as well as capacity building and programme management. This approach to building awareness of challenges faced and co-creating solutions with a set of stakeholders while keeping the marginalised and underserved at the centre generates the need for further social innovation – be it in developing new products, services or market access mechanisms – that leads to newer forms of collective organisations and wider social practices. New challenges and practices to address them create social changes that seek to alter the pattern of resource allocation and power relations in society. The emphasis on social demands from underprivileged communities, problem-solving with multiple stakeholders and the requirement to achieve social change are some of the factors that distinguish social innovation from other forms of innovation.

The study of the mechanisms by which potential capabilities can be transformed into realised capabilities among stakeholders, including the government and communities, can provide a deeper understanding of the process of social innovation. Social innovation ecosystems unleash the power of individual and collective creativity, learning and adaptation in a variety of contexts that, in turn, lead to building and sustaining capabilities and social realisations (Nussbaum & Sen, 1993). This creativity can range from thinking critically to combining unrelated processes to enhance the social impact.

This chapter demonstrates how social innovation in urban sanitation has embraced the idea of organisation building for the urban poor, especially to address the social inequality in accessing urban sanitation services, including the lack of safety and dignity for sanitation workers. The need to be organised along the lines of social, locational, caste or gender identities has often foregrounded social innovation in urban sanitation, at the local and national levels. There is a link between how urban sanitation as a civic service (and right) functions in society and how society is organised, facilitating access to safe, reliable and sustainable sanitation facilities and services. How marginal groups face the challenges of social isolation related to sanitation and overcome them are important sites for social innovation.

A common feature is that some stakeholders act as catalysts to drive change by organising groups at various political, social or even policy levels. The organisation of groups and communities, the building of communication channels between privileged and disfavoured citizens within urban society, and the creation of people's democracy at the local level (e.g., neighbourhoods, small communities, and groups of homeless, unemployed and informal workers, among others) are factors of innovation in social relations.

At the core of any social innovation lies its communitarian approach. Community participation is a powerful organising ideal that fosters more equitable development in and of communities. It can contribute to local development planning and design. It is crucial to facilitate processes that empower people to come together, understand their realities, articulate their needs and demands, formulate solutions and take collective decisions.

The history of organisation building for participation in state-sponsored development programmes began in the 1970s with international aid agencies and grassroots activists putting demands on the governments of developing countries to make community participation a part of social development programmes. Participation emerged from the margin of development discourse in the 1970s with the assertion of the Basic Needs Approach by the International Labour Organisation (ILO). Cornwall (2000) outlined the arguments made for participation in the 1960s and 1970s into three distinct tributaries – participation 'for' the people, 'by' the people and 'with' the people. The 'for' the people argument centred on the necessity of participation in increasing or improving the efficiency and effectiveness of the development projects – an argument that has survived over time and is still at the centre stage of the participation debate (Tandon & Kak, 2007). The 'by' the people stream of thought looked at participation from the standpoint of a struggle for 'right, recognition and more equitable distribution of resources' (Cornwall, 2000). 'The "with" the people view of participation was grounded in the belief that people cannot be developed; they can only develop themselves' (Neyere, 1973; Hall et al., 1982).

Rahman (1982) made a distinction between 'participatory development' and 'people's self-development'. The mainstream discourse saw participation as a means to involve people in activities initiated by the development agencies or the state. In contrast, people's self-development approach considered participation as a process of collective action and mobilisation that could lead to self-reliant development and the capacity to negotiate new terms with those in power, including the state (Stiefel & Wolfe, 1994).

Since the 1990s, community participation has come to be recognised as a key ingredient in sanitation programmes. There have been two approaches that proliferated – the first, where projects created structures of the beneficiary communities in the form of committees to facilitate participation; the second, where external non-governmental organisations (NGOs) were involved in eliciting community participation in projects. Despite such strides, organisation building has remained difficult due to reasons that range from a top-down attitude of government bureaucracy, and the additional time required for building community participation structures, to conflicts of interest within communities. In current times, governments are seeking active support from NGOs in the form of partnerships to set up community institutions and mobilise community participation for the effective delivery of services. It is pertinent to note in this context that much service delivery to the poor happens only when there is a clear will demonstrated by the government. Community-based institutions take up the role of information dissemination, articulation of collective demand, collaboration and negotiation with the government for demand fulfilment and even assertion of interest in situations where the government agencies ignore some issues.

This chapter aims to shed light on this aspect of social innovation by explaining how organisation building has been approached in seven cases. Social innovation in this context seems to play an important role in connecting people and governments with civil society affecting this innovation by way of education, enhancement programmes, grassroots empowerment, etc. Subsequent sections of the chapter discuss cases where social innovation was engineered in urban sanitation by bringing people and communities together at small and large scales. The idea is to foreground organisation building as one of the key elements of the social innovation process, especially in urban sanitation.

## 3. MOBILISING SANITATION WORKERS TO END MANUAL SCAVENGING

Social innovations related to a much-neglected issue of manual scavenging have been spearheaded by the Safai Karmachari Andolan (SKA), which has evolved as an all-India movement committed to the abolition of the dehumanising practice of manual scavenging and dignified rehabilitation of those who have undertaken this work of physically removing untreated human excreta using the most basic tools. SKA started its work in the 1980s, committed exclusively to the issues of sanitation workers. In doing so, SKA brought the human perspective of sanitation to the forefront. The story of the evolution of the SKA into a people's movement is itself the story of social innovation at work. The organisational values of human dignity, self-respect and equality encompass their work and percolate into the social innovations it has led.

SKA classifies '*safai karmachari*' or sanitation workers into three groups: (i) manual scavengers, (ii) sewerage workers and (iii) septic tank workers. SKA estimates that 98 percent of manual scavengers are women as men generally work as sewerage workers or septic tank workers. Although the foremost focus was establishing the rights of manual scavengers, SKA expressed its commitments to all those engaged in 'unclean' occupations. SKA promotes the idea of the least possible human intervention in all these three above types of sanitation work. By bringing this social issue to the forefront and insisting that urban sanitation is not just about waste management and toilets but equally about manual scavenging, SKA generated its unique brand of social innovation by organising, documenting and bringing this issue back into the consciousness of decision-makers and civil society.

Through its different interventions, SKA envisages highlighting the struggles and building solidarity to reclaim the dignity, equality and human personhood of the *safai karmachari*. Furthermore, it envisions that by eradicating manual scavenging, SKA will break the link imposed by the caste system between birth and dehumanising occupations. SKA strives for the liberation and rehabilitation of all persons engaged in manual scavenging across India from their caste-based hereditary and inhuman occupation. The SKA's major focus is to organise and mobilise the community around the issues of dignity and rights, accompanied by strategic advocacy and legal interventions. Since it represents a national movement, SKA encompasses both the rural and urban in terms of its presence. Its network is present in 25 states across India with more than 6,000 volunteers. The thematic areas of its activities mainly revolve around advocacy, networking and coalition building, rehabilitation of present manual scavengers alongside facilitating education, skill training and employment of youth from the communities. A major portion of SKA's interventions deals with the prevention of the death of *safai karmachari* through awareness generation and facilitation of families of 'sanitation victims' for compensation through proper channels, besides advocacy for innovative solutions in the sanitation sector.

### Box 3.1 SKA and Bhim Yatra

One of the most successful campaigns of SKA has been the Bhim Yatra. It was launched as a country-wide march to diffuse the idea of the social innovation pioneered by SKA. The *yatra* symbolised a journey of pain and anguish to tell the country and the government to 'stop killing us' in dry latrines, sewers and septic tanks. The Bhim Yatra, according to SKA, symbolised a journey of intolerance of violence, discrimination and violation of constitutional and fundamental rights. It was envisaged to spread Ambedkar's ideas of social justice, liberty, equality and fraternity. The *yatra* was launched from Vishwa Yuvak Kendra, New Delhi, on 10 December 2015 and set off from Dibrugarh, Assam, on 11 December 2015. The journey moved continuously for 125 days from one state to another, covering 500 districts, and ended on 13 April 2016 in Delhi, on the eve of the 125th birth anniversary of Dr BR Ambedkar.

Although executed in 2015, the foundations for such a march like the Bhim Yatra could be traced back further. Since 1982, SKA has been raising its voice against the discrimination of sanitation workers. SKA has organised, mobilised and campaigned against the atrocity and for the discontinuation of dry latrines and its link with the dehumanising occupation of manual scavenging. In 1993, the parliament passed 'The Employment of Manual Scavengers and Construction of Dry Latrines (Prohibition) Act'. The Act made a provision for imprisonment of up to one year and/or a fine of Rs 2,000 to the violators. However, this law has never led to convictions during the past couple of decades. The government made repeated promises to eliminate the heinous practice of manual scavenging. In 2003, SKA filed a Public Interest Litigation (PIL) in the Supreme Court of India. A total denial from the state governments about the existence of manual scavenging was followed by partial admission when SKA produced photographic evidence. The Supreme Court imposed compliance to some extent. In 2007, with the solidarity and support from civil society groups and public leaders, SKA launched the Action 2010 campaign to end manual scavenging by December 2010, but it was all in vain. Hence, SKA started the historical bus *yatra* in October 2010. This *Samajik Parivartan Yatra*, which was the first of its kind, journeyed the entire country. Many women and men engaged in manual scavenging work came out and led the *yatra*, which ended in New Delhi with a mammoth public meeting.

Apart from these social actions, SKA has also submitted memorandums to the President, Prime Minister, ministries, statutory bodies and the National Advisory Council (NAC) (an advisory committee formed in 2004 by the previous union government to advise the then Prime Minister). The memorandums demanded the implementation of the 1993 Act and a rehabilitation package. The NAC passed a resolution on 23 October 2010 to end manual scavenging by 31 March 2012. After the *yatra*, the then Minister of Social Justice and Empowerment invited SKA for a discussion. SKA submitted the nationwide data collected during the *yatra*. Following that meeting, the Ministry of Social Justice and Empowerment convened the national consultation on 24–25 January 2011, which resulted in the setting up of four task forces – to review the Act, conduct a national survey and revise the rehabilitation package and sanitation solutions. The President of India in her speech to the parliament at the start of the budget session in March 2012, announced the draft of a new bill for the prohibition of manual scavenging. The Government of India passed the new 'Prohibition of Employment as Manual Scavengers and their Rehabilitation Act 2013' in September 2013 and issued a Government Notification in December 2013.

## 4. AMPLIFYING THE VOICES OF WOMEN

The vulnerabilities that women and girls living in slums and informal settlements may face every day when making their sanitation choices are probably the most profound of the gender inequalities that occur in urban settings (Chaplin, 2017). It has also been often highlighted in the literature that the vulnerability of women and girls to gender-based violence increased in situations where they were accessing water and sanitation. Of the many organisations that have worked towards alleviating this vulnerability, Gramalaya has been at the forefront now for more than three decades. Using the new spaces offered by the Swachh Bharat Mission (SBM) of 2014, which linked urban sanitation with international development priorities, Gramalaya has enhanced its role as a catalyst in the urban sanitation sector by stepping up its earlier engagement in the informal settlements of Tiruchirappalli (Trichy), Tamil Nadu.

The social innovation approach of Gramalaya consisted of adapting the lessons learnt from its long engagement in providing sanitation to marginalised communities. The innovation did not involve a new idea but rather improvised an existing idea to meet the unmet sanitation needs in the urban sector. The highlight of its social innovation was how it used the expertise it had acquired over three decades of work in rural sanitation to deepen its urban work once the framework for urban interventions was set by the SBM. In line with its community-based approach to urban sanitation, Gramalaya formed the Association of Water, Sanitation and Hygiene (AWASH).

---

**Box 3.2 AWASH Committee**

Each AWASH committee consists of ten male and ten female members and has an advisor. The field representative of Gramalaya acts as the secretary of the committee. The committee members are provided handholding training for data collection, IEC activities and basic technical know-how related to different types of toilets, alongside toilet usage practices. Furthermore, they were provided information on health and hygiene practices, including hand washing. The community members are trained to handle funds provided for the construction of toilets through training in book keeping and basic accountancy. An important outcome of the social innovation that was set in motion by Gramalaya's work in urban sanitation was handing over the toilets to the women Self-Help Federation (SHF) after the construction and refurbishment of community toilets by the Municipal Corporation, thereby bringing in women as important stakeholders in the social project.

---

Gramalaya's interventions have had a ripple impact by generating confidence among women and bringing them into decision-making roles on other issues of slum welfare as well. Overall, it combined the technical innovations in toilet models developed by its Centre for Toilet Technology and Training with community-managed microfinance for different sanitation models with a child and woman-friendly approach that encourages margin-alised communities to invest in creating a context where toilets will not only be constructed in urban slums but also used and managed at the local level, making the community the primary stakeholder in the process. In 2000, supported by WaterAid, Gramalaya undertook the construction, renova-tion, operation and management of community toilets in Tiruchirappalli city (Trichy). The existing community toilets managed by the Trichy City Corporation (TCC) were not in use as they remained dirty, unhygienic and dysfunctional. Through a process of community participation facilitated by Gramalaya, women took charge of community toilet complexes (CTCs) promoted by a partnership between the Municipal Corporation, commu-nities and the NGOs. Gramalaya formed self-help groups (SHGs) in each informal settlement, where each SHG had members of 10–15 women. All SHGs within an informal settlement constituted a Sanitation and Hygiene Education – Team (SHE-Team). The SHE-Teams assumed the responsibili-ties of planning, implementing, monitoring and maintaining the entire sani-tation programme, including raising awareness within the community and ensuring that people move away from the practice of open defecation (OD). On average, members of half the households in a community were part of the SHGs, thereby ensuring that half the community was directly involved in issues related to sanitation in an informal settlement. The Community Toilet Blocks in Tiruchirappalli provide a clean environment, child-friendly seats, disabled-friendly seats, facilities for hygienic disposal of cloth used as sanitary pads during menstruation and hand-washing facilities (basins with soap) in most Women's Action for Village Empowerment (or WAVE, a network of SHGs) supported toilets. These toilets have ten seats for men and ten for women. They also offer bathing and clothes washing facilities.

Another case where organisation building among women has led to better outcomes is that of Project Nirmal in Odisha, implemented by the Centre for Policy Research (CPR) and Practical Action (PA) in collabo-ration with the State Government of Odisha. This has purposefully tar-geted women to come forward and be recognised by the communities to represent them. Besides women who have been active in the community, the inclusion of *Anganwadi* (Early Childhood Care Centre) and ASHA (Accredited Social Health Activists) workers as SHGs have expanded the space for women in the Slum Sanitation Committees (SSC) that have been formed under Project Nirmal. With time, it has been realised that women can be better functionaries as SSC members for practical reasons. While men often go out to work, women stay at home and, thus, are aware of local sanitation issues in more nuanced ways than men. All the SSCs that were studied under Project Nirmal were reported to have women as active members and leaders who both work within the community to spread awareness and information and address the service delivery issues with the municipality and other government officials. Male members pitch in when required. For example, they can go to fetch mosquito oil from the municipality office or when their support is required in a difficult situation, such as in the event of someone falling sick and needing to be taken to the hospital. Though the latter is not a mandatory function of SSCs, they extend support to people from within their informal settlements during times of crisis.

The stories of both Project Nirmal and Gramalaya go to show that putting women at the forefront is critical. Women have been traditionally responsible for cleanliness and sanitation of the private space of households, but SSCs and SHE Toilets in their different ways have brought women into the public space. On the one hand, it shoulders more responsibility on them with extra work, while on the other, it brings them into decision-making positions that have traditionally been denied to them. In the latter role, they expand their identities and roles beyond the confines of homes and families and emerge as community representatives, leaders and managers. Women filling and occupying public spaces are not only a source of self-empowerment, but they also empower women as a collective.

## 5. WORKING WITH THE STATE TO ACHIEVE SANITATION GOALS: URBAN POOR AND LOW-INCOME GROUPS

The core principles of any social innovation in urban sanitation have to be about reaching those whom benefits and developmental programmes hardly reach and thereafter organising this unorganised sector irrespective of caste, ethnicity, religion, gender or economic status. To do this, a right-based approach must be followed, which is 'biased' towards the underprivileged, such as the urban poor and low-income groups, and works through advocacy and implementation of existing laws and programmes for realising their rights. The urban poor is a heterogeneous category that has been both explored and addressed through various social innovations by several civil society organisations. The concerns of this group have been taken into consideration in many urban development programmes and policies, and urban sanitation is no exception to this. In the context of this development, it is only obvious that social innovations in the field of urban sanitation follow this route. The low-income group is another heterogeneous category of several sub-groups, namely vendors, hawkers, rag pickers and other individuals engaged in lesser-paid informal activities. Ensuring their access to safe and sustainable sanitation has been a major challenge for the state. This challenge is aggravated by the lack of infrastructure in and around their dwellings. Due to inadequate housing facilities and unsafe work conditions, providing them with clean and affordable sanitation becomes both crucial and tough. To ensure that the rights of the underprivileged are provided for, it is important for civil society organisations to actively engage the service provider at local government, state and national levels to influence funding, implementation, programme and policy.

## *Engaged citizens, responsive city initiative of PRIA*

One of the most successful outcomes of such associations can be found in the case of the **Engaged Citizens, Responsive City (ECRC)** initiative of Participatory Research in Asia (PRIA). The key objective of the ECRC initiative was to strengthen the civil societies of the urban poor and enable them to meaningfully participate in and influence the planning and monitoring of sanitation services in Indian cities. The project began in 2016 and focused on three Smart Cities and their informal settlements – Ajmer in Rajasthan, Jhansi in Uttar Pradesh and Muzaffarpur in Bihar.

It focused on mobilising and organising the urban poor to counter the 'informality' attached to their existence and the services they received, but most importantly it 'mapped' them and their settlements. ECRC focused on a four-phase action strategy wherein it created an environment that enabled change and action: (a) **information** or the understanding and exchanging of information about the conditions; (b) **awareness** or building individual and collective awareness of the hurdles and opportunities around the conditions; (c) **mobilisation** or organising communities to unite for a goal and (d) **action** or jointly undertaking processes to achieve the goal.

PRIA, along with the local ward councillors, began with mapping and updating lists of informal settlements to counter the lack of authentic data regarding urban poor settlements. Building relations and involving the local councillor were essential to the credibility of the processes with the community. The mapping process physically identified and plotted the settlements in the city, and their basic information, irrespective of their legal status (or lack thereof) recognised by the city authorities. This was because information on informal settlements available with city authorities/agencies is either not updated or not inclusive of all informal settlements. This excludes large clusters of communities from consideration during city planning or development. Consequently, people living in these unrecorded settlements are always at the risk of eviction and lack basic amenities like water supply, sanitation, electricity and other services.

Apart from creating an authentic database of those living in the city, the mapping process also created an opportunity to initiate interactions with the communities living in these settlements. Focus Group Discussions, transect walks and informal engagements helped identify active citizens and leaders in the community as well as other community-based organisations (CBOs) and social institutions that were dormant or active in the settlements.

The mapping process brought out the discrepancies between the number of informal settlements that existed on the ground and other secondary records. For example, in Ajmer, the number of informal settlements as reported by municipal records was 83; however, the mapping and listing exercise physically identified as many as 125 informal settlements with the help of residents. In Jhansi, 75 settlements were identified on the ground against the city authority's record of only 57.

These discrepancies, along with information on relevant stakeholders secured through formal and informal community interactions, helped secure significant data and access to officials from Municipal Corporations, ward councillors, former councillors, community leaders, various CBOs, etc. To sustain these interactions, PRIA simultaneously held meetings with other citizen groups, media people concerned about city and sanitation issues, and active NGOs in all three cities. This was essential to build an environment where municipal official stakeholders were beginning to be held accountable by civil society groups for the identified lags in sanitation and other civic services.

These interactions gathered enough consensus and raised awareness about the need for informal settlement dwellers to organise themselves into Settlement Improvement Committees (SICs). SICs were representative bodies established with nominated residents of the informal settlement. Each SIC had a total of 8–15 members. The project had made a conscious emphasis on the greater involvement of youth and women as members and leaders of these committees. SICs acted as bridges between the service providers and the community. They worked as organisations that spoke in unison about the communities' needs and rights. They were the focal points through which external stakeholders could connect with the communities. Unlike other interventions that approach women and youth empowerment by constituting exclusive groups, ECRC focused on integrating women and youth leadership into the intervention as a whole, building their capacity at par with men and the elderly. It was also essential to identify youth leadership as they would be the future of the settlements, and it was important to empower them as responsible citizens. It was also important to address issues related to sanitation, health and education affecting children and youth in the informal settlements to sustain SICs and their goals.

A significant part of maintaining the momentum of the SICs was scaling it up from the bottom (or settlements) to the city level – an aspect missing in most developmental interventions. While each SIC implemented something transformative in their neighbourhoods after harnessing the survey findings, their presence at the city level was missing. As the SICs launched into the surveys and associated actions, the need for a city-level SIC institution was felt. Such an institution would influence city-wide decision-making processes and support individual SICs. Thus, SIC members began building their organisations towards an SIC Forum – a city-level network of SICs. The idea and purpose of the SIC Forum were to expand the resource and network bases and the bargaining power of the urban poor at the city level. It created a multistakeholder interface with city associations, such as the citizen forum (a mixed association of residents from informal settlements, middle-income colonies, professional associations and other civil society groups catalysed by the ECRC initiative), academic institutes, traders, markets and professional associations, resident welfare associations (RWAs), and connected them to individual SICs. Such an elaborate network increased its credibility and enabled its members to address development challenges beyond sanitation in the future. Launched in the three cities mentioned earlier, the SIC Forum also focused on equal leadership of men, women and youth representing various informal settlements. The PRIA team intensified engagement with its urban poor stakeholders by organising exposure visits to partner cities. This facilitated the exchange of experiences among members from various SICs and helped them initiate dialogues and facilitate negotiations with city authorities and other stakeholders. The forums continue to help communities articulate their needs and facilitate their participation in city-level sanitation planning, implementation and monitoring.

By organising the urban poor, the ECRC initiative brought critical information and awareness among communities, generated increased demand for sanitation services and other entitlements and increased responsiveness from the municipalities.

### Organising collective action by Nidan

Another successful example of organising collective action on urban sanitation is the work of Nidan with hawkers and vendors at their homes (given the transient nature of their workplaces) through the formation of the National Association of Street Vendors of India (NASVI) in 1998. By actively engaging in the same slum community on multiple issues and working at a 'pan ward' and 'pan city' approach, Nidan has successfully aligned and leveraged multiple schemes and developmental programmes of the service providers and helped the urban poor access their entitlements from local and state governments. Nidan works with people in the informal sector to assist them in accessing a range of developmental services, including assisting informal settlement dwellers in procuring sanitation services. Its Urban Sanitation Programme is a community-led intervention that leverages its existing workers' groups and processes, including educational meetings, resource centres and schools, to spread sanitation and hygiene awareness. This knowledge is used to influence the government to design policies that are appropriate for existing urban conditions. Since the workplace of urban hawkers and vendors is not fixed, the strategic decision was to collectivise them instead at their places of residence. Consequently, Nidan started its interventions on shelter, livelihood, health and education in informal settlements and homeless hamlets that are 'home' to these unorganised workers. How the hawkers and vendors, who are integral to India's urban landscape, were brought into the sanitation project by harnessing their networks to raise awareness about toilet usage lies at the heart of Nidan's social innovation approach.

### Alliance building by SPARC, NSDF and MM

The Society for Promotion of Area Resource Centre (SPARC) formed an alliance with the National Slum Dwellers Federation (NSDF) and Mahila

Milan (MM), which helped in reconfiguring the relationships between the city government, civil society and communities by turning them into partners. Starting in Mumbai, innovations in organisation building led to the city government recognising the capacity of community organisations to develop their own solutions, which was supported by local civil society organisations (CSOs). In the case of SPARC, the division of roles was also clear with city authorities who changed their role from being a toilet provider to the one setting standards, funding the capital cost of construction and providing water and electricity. The CSOs and community organisations designed, built and maintained the toilet blocks.

Over the years, this alliance has institutionalised its methodologies for organising the urban poor, which are often referred to as 'rituals'. These are discussed in detail below.

### Surveys and enumerations

A very powerful instrument of the alliance process is the poor collecting data about themselves. The alliance facilitates three types of data collection. One is of developing profiles of the informal settlements that helps the city authorities and communities know all informal settlements in the city. In addition, it involves collecting household and individual data to deepen and sharpen household and individual identities within neighbourhoods. All the data are then integrated with the city planning processes.

### Women's participation and savings groups in informal settlements

Unlike other micro-credit movements where women savings groups serve mainly economic functions and become financial delivery mechanisms, within the alliance daily savings is a means for women to initially pool very small amounts of money and lend to each other during crises or immediate needs. To collect the money, account for it and create lending rules, they begin their journey into financial management and trust building. Gradually, as their process begins to mature, they begin to receive external money to slowly expand their capacity to lend.

### Precedent-setting and partnerships for change

Precedent-setting begins when discussions are initiated about how to create something that works for the poor but is not yet accepted by the city government. The alliance systematically identifies practices that make complete sense to the urban poor and invite government officials and technical professionals to see and recognise the essence of this collective action. When that is accepted, it is promoted as a precedent so that the multiplication of the act produces its acceptability.

### Developing voice and advocacy externally

The alliance sees the issues of advocacy deeply wrapped within its ongoing pursuit of making cities inclusive and work for all. The alliance leadership believes that designing solutions and alternatives is vital for social movements. These solutions and strategies are the physical manifestations of the demands the social movements of the poor make on themselves. If sanitation is a crisis for the urban poor, they focus on creating a strategy to highlight its value to them, seek a wide consensus about it within their own organisations, and develop the confidence to start seeking the involvement of the state and other actors in addressing this challenge.

### The network's engagement with the state and professionals

The alliance believes that the state has a responsibility to its poorest citizens and there is a need to change the current asymmetric relationship to one of engagement and ultimately of partnership. The alliance members often invite the professionals and politicians in large gatherings of the federated communities. The organised management of the event, clear and simple representation, and sharing of possible alternatives to a problem by the community are in stark contrast to the accusatory and confrontational responses the professionals or politicians sometimes experience elsewhere. The alliance leaders also invited politicians, administrators and professionals to accompany them on learning exchanges to see how a similar problem was solved elsewhere through engagement and negotiation, and how it was good for the city as well as for the poor. The strategy was to see what was possible. Today, peer dialogues between ministers, mayors, administrators and informal settlement dwellers occur during these same visits.

---

**Box 3.3 The Alliance of SPARC, National Slum Dwellers Federation and Mahila Milan**

In Pune, a partnership between the municipal government, NGOs and CBOs built more than 400 community toilet blocks between 1999 and 2001, which greatly improved sanitation for more than half a million people. They also demonstrated the potential of municipal–community partnerships to improve conditions for low-income groups. In 1999, the Municipal Commissioner of Pune sought to increase the scale of public toilet construction and ensure that more appropriate toilets were built. Advertisements were placed in newspapers, inviting NGOs to bid for toilet construction projects. SPARC was one of the NGOs to receive the contract, working with the National Slum Dwellers Federation (NSDF) and Mahila Milan (MM). The alliance of these three institutions had been working in Pune for several years, supporting a vibrant savings and credit movement among women slum dwellers. Their work also included experiments with community toilets. Now the alliance became one of the principal contractors and constructed 114 toilet blocks (with more than 2,000 toilet seats and 500 children's toilet seats). The alliance designed and evaluated the project, while the city provided the capital and the communities developed the capacity for management and maintenance. Between 1999 and 2001, more toilets were constructed and more funds allocated than in the previous 30 years. Overall, more than 400 toilet blocks were built with over 10,000 seats, at a cost of around Rs 40 crore.

### Social mobilisation by CURE

The Centre for Urban and Regional Excellence's (CURE's) work in projects like the JJ Colony in Noida, Kuchpura in Agra and at Savda Ghevra, Safeda Basti and Nepali Camp in Delhi are examples of how social mobilisation can help in increasing communities' access to toilets, septic tanks and sewer systems. By working for the development of low-income communities in urban informal settlements, CURE has achieved last-mile connectivity as far as sanitation services are concerned for the communities they work with. CURE uses its in-house experts such as planners, engineers and architects to ensure that the solutions are scientifically sound. A significant part of CURE's work involves building infrastructure such as toilets, drainage and sewer systems, for the communities. According to CURE, the core of its social innovation approach is the belief that transformation is possible only when communities 'un-think, re-imagine, innovate and de-engineer solutions' that integrate people into city development processes.

### Box 3.4 Centre for Urban and Regional Excellence (CURE)

CURE, in partnership with communities in Safeda Basti and Savda Ghevra, Delhi, successfully implemented a project called, 'Connecting the Disconnect: Realising Household Toilets in Safeda Basti'. The project involved working towards an innovative and sustainable sanitation solution where people were in partnership with the local service provider, in this case, the Delhi Urban Shelter Improvement Board (DUSIB), Delhi Jal Board (DJB) and East Delhi Municipal Corporation (EDMC). CURE conducted a Total Sanitation Survey (TSS) and obtained permission from the DJB to connect the settlement to the main sewer line. CURE laid a sewer line under the main street of the settlement, which was then connected to individual houses. It made sure that the community was involved in all stages of the project (planning, implementation and monitoring) so that the people would have a sense of ownership of the built infrastructure.

By making the people primary stakeholders, CURE not only developed capacities in communities but also empowered them to make decisions that suited them most. In these projects, the communities have successfully carried on even after the organisation's active involvement had ended. Having targeted community mobilisation and empowerment, CURE was able to build people's confidence, resulting in a deeper impact related to behaviour change.

## 6. CONCLUSION

Organising communities and ensuring community participation can be most rewarding when it brings people and local governments together to discuss problems, explore options and choose best-fit solutions for their area's development. As elaborated in the case studies above, participation helps people, including the poor, apply their local wisdom, bring in value from self-organised networks, overcome personal differences and collaborate in reshaping their environments. At the core of any social innovation, the approach is that it brings about a process of change to meet critical needs. For such changes to meet urban sanitation needs, they have to be envisioned by utilising the knowledge of the community who are the end-users of the services and organising them to get involved in solution-making and in delivering these services. After all, people and communities are the most important stakeholders, and they have to play the most important role in any social innovation that is to affect their lives.

Creating and strengthening the interface between governance and community is helpful to both – government agencies get to know about community issues and people get to know the agencies and officials responsible for sanitation services. Regular interaction among stakeholders eliminates mutual distrust and suspicion. It instils confidence among people and a sense of responsibility among service providers. Collaboration and partnership with concerned agencies with a sanitation mandate are important to engage in the governance processes. Identifying the agencies and forging and negotiating collaboration are of vital importance in making the delivery of sanitation services collaborative, efficient and regular. Almost all the organisations mentioned in this chapter have had stakeholder engagement as an important component of their organisation-building strategy. SPARC in Pune, CURE in Delhi and Gramalaya in Trichy worked in close collaboration with government agencies in promoting community-led CTCs. The ECRC initiative of PRIA facilitated a culture of dialogue between the organised community and local governance institutions based on data and evidence generated by the community itself.

Generating and strengthening collective demand through community platforms create collective strength, voice, strategy and leadership that are required to put pressure on service delivery. Social innovation in the field of organisation building has helped people access other services besides sanitation, such as electricity, social security and housing. Pointing this out is crucial because one of the features of service delivery in India has been that even though government programmes do intend to include the poor, the services either do not reach them or reach them insufficiently due to the lack of better information or contact. In light of this reality, bringing people together and enabling them to organise themselves can prove to be an effective strategy for addressing the existing inequalities in urban sanitation services.

Collectivisation, participation and improved dialogue and understanding between the public agencies, marginalised communities, CSOs and other stakeholders have two-way benefits for improving sanitation. The first has been discussed in this chapter. The second – that of the need for collectivisation and participation – is discussed in the next chapter.

# 4 Sustainable Behaviour Change in the Community

## 1. INTRODUCTION

This chapter deals with social innovations adopted in development communication for urban sanitation. It explores various innovations primarily facilitated by civil society organisations (CSOs) in the urban sanitation space to encourage behaviour change in communities and other stakeholders. Swachh Bharat Mission – Urban (SBM-U), popularly known as the CLEAN India Campaign, launched in 2014 by the Government of India (GOI) is seen as the largest behaviour change campaign in the history of urban development programmes in India. While the programme's main focus was to end open defecation (OD) in rural and urban India, solid and liquid waste management (SLWM) also became a central focus to curb environmental pollution for improved health outcomes.

Sanitation is just not about toilets but also about the safe containment of faeces, safe emptying, transportation and safe treatment of the faecal waste to curb environmental pollution. India's greater reliance on onsite sanitation systems (60 percent of urban households use some form of an onsite sanitation system) brings to the fore the importance of Faecal Sludge and Septage Management (FSSM). By 2017, the GOI developed a National Policy on FSSM, followed by many state governments focusing on FSSM. Another national flagship programme, Atal Mission for Rejuvenation and Urban Transformation (AMRUT), contemporary to the SBM, supported the state governments to undertake FSSM in various Indian cities.

SBM-U and the National Policy on FSSM emphasised awareness generation and behaviour change campaigns acknowledging that technological innovations and investments in infrastructure can only sustain with strategic communication approaches. The communication campaigns in India around FSSM began to be mainstreamed post-2016–2017, with an increasing focus on the management of faecal sludge.

This chapter traces the meaning and evolution of development communication, the approaches and methods used in development communication and its adoption in the urban sanitation ecosystem.

DOI: 10.4324/9781003197102-4

## 2. DEVELOPMENT COMMUNICATION: MEANING AND EVOLUTION

Development communication has always remained a powerful approach for reaching out to people with messages and information so that attitudinal and behaviour change can be effected to bring about desired social change.

Development communication involves the strategic use of communication for the alleviation of social problems in evolving societies (Wilkins, 2007). It has been defined by many scholars to include the practice of systematically applying the processes, strategies and principles of communication to bring about positive social change. The term 'development communication' was first coined in 1972 by Nora C Quebral, who defines the field as 'the art and science of human communication linked to a society's planned transformation from a state of poverty to one of dynamic socioeconomic growth that makes for greater equity and the larger unfolding of individual potential' (Quebral, 2001).

Wilkins and Mody (2001) define development communication as a process of strategic intervention towards social change initiated by institutions and communities. Jayaweera (1987) conceptualises it as the communication strategies of a whole society or the communication component of a national development plan. Even during the emergence of the dominant development paradigm, communication involving community participation formed a very important facet in the promotion of sustainable development (Bessette & Rajasunderam, 1996; Cadiz, 1994; Craig & Mayo, 1995). Corroborating this, Manyozo (2006) defines modern-day development communication as describing a group of method-driven and theory-based praxes that employ participatory foreground and backdrop communication tools in strengthening community decision-making processes and structures to improve livelihoods and promote social justice. Table 4.1 describes approaches to development communication by six schools as described by Manyozo.

After World War II, with the establishment of Bretton Woods Institutes, the focus was to rebuild underdeveloped nations. Western countries tended to locate the problem in underdeveloped nations without acknowledging the unequal relationship that existed between these nations and more powerful economies. It was assumed that the Western models of development were appropriate for all parts of the world. The failure of many development projects in the 1960s led to the reconceptualisation of its top-down methods. The Bretton Woods School has reviewed its approaches over the years and has been the most dynamic in testing and adopting new approaches and methodologies. The World Bank currently defines development communication as the 'integration of strategic communication in development projects' based on a clear understanding of indigenous realities (Manyozo, 2006).

The Latin American school inspired by Paulo Freire's work used participatory and educational rural radio approaches to empower the marginalised.

*Table 4.1* Approaches to development communication

| | | |
|---|---|---|
| 1940 **The Latin America School**<br>(Radio *Sutatenza* for rural education; Miners' Radio Network in Colombia; Television and radio entertainment education)<br>*Theorists:* **Acción Cultural Popular (ACPO)**, Luis Ramiro Beltrán, Juan Díaz Bordenave, Miguel Sabido, Paulo Freire, Jose Barrientos | Earliest models for participatory broadcasting efforts around the world. In the 1960s, Paulo Freire's theories of critical pedagogy and Miguel Sabido's enter-educate method became important elements of the Latin American development communication scene. In the 1990s, technological advances facilitated social change and development | Rural radio approaches to empower the marginalised |
| 1950 **The Bretton Woods School**<br>*Theorist:* Everett Rogers, Daniel Lerner, Wilbur Schramm, Jan Servaes, Steeves & Melkote, UNESCO, WB, UNDP, FAO, John Hopkins Centre for Communication Programs, SADC Centre of Communication for Development, IDRC | Economic strategies outlined in the Marshall Plan after World War II, and the establishment of the Bretton Woods system, the World Bank and the International Monetary Fund in 1944. Production and planting of development in indigenous societies | Use of mass communication to address problems in underdeveloped nations. Today, the school's largest institution, the World Bank, conceptualises devcom as an 'integration of strategic communication in development projects' that is based on a clear understanding of 'indigenous realities' |
| 1950 **The Los Baños School**<br>(Development broadcasting; agricultural development communication).<br>*Theorists:* Felix Librero, Alexander Flor, Ely Gomez, Nora Quebral, Juan Jamias, Madeline Suva, Virginia Samonte, Communication Foundation for Asia, Philippine Press Institute, International Rice Research Institute | Evolved to include development broadcasting and telecommunications, development journalism, educational communication, science communication, strategic communication and health communication | |

| 1960 | **The African School** (Rural radio; Theatre for development) *Theorists*: Penina Mlama, Christopher Kamlongera, Zakes Mda, Robert MacLaren, Ngugi wa Thiong'o, Mapopa Mtonga, Derek Mulenga, David Kerr, Jean-Pierre Ilboudo, Center for Rural Broadcasting Studies of Ouagadougou (CIERRO) | In the 1990s, the FAO project, 'Communication for Development in Southern Africa', was a pioneer in supporting and enhancing development projects and programmes through the use of participatory communication approaches. An innovative methodology known as Participatory Rural Communication Appraisal (PRCA) was in place and is still widely used today in various projects around the world | Use of theatre |
| 1970 | **The Indian School** (Radio/television for rural development, development journalism) *Theorists*: Mehra Masani, George Verghese Keval Kumar, University of Poona, Joseph Velacherry, Delhi University, University of Kerala | Community development projects initiated by the Union Government in the 1950s | Rural radio broadcasts in Marathi, Hindi, Gujarati and Kannada |
| 1980 | **Post-Freire School: Participatory Development Communication** (Communication for social change/development – visual anthropology, community theatre, public journalism, radio for development, development radio broadcasting) *Theorists*: UPLB College of Development Communication, IDRC, FAO Communication Project, UNESCO, Rockefeller Foundation, Ford Foundation, World Bank | Involvement of the community in development efforts, collaboration between First World and Third World development communication organisations | Community at the heart of development communication; use of participatory tools and methods, including theatre and radio broadcasting |

*Source*: Adapted from Manyozo (2006)

The history of organised development communication in India goes back to rural radio broadcasts of the 1940s in regional languages such as Hindi, Marathi, Gujarati and Kannada. After independence, India witnessed early organised experiments in development communication with community development projects initiated by the GOI in the 1950s. While field publicity was given due importance for person-to-person communication – because the rural literacy level was very low – radio played an equally important role in reaching the masses.

Historically, the aim of development communication has been information-based mass communication, proposing to use the potential of information and communication to enhance the process of socioeconomic development. Its purposes included informing, creating awareness, educating and enlightening the people so they could better their lives. In developing countries, interpersonal communication mechanisms have been more effective, based on participation rather than mass media campaigns. Increasingly, development programmes focused on self-development at the village and urban neighbourhood levels as well as the importance of small, local-level discussion groups have been recognised – e.g., mothers' clubs in Korea, farmers' associations in Taiwan and radio listening clubs in Tanzania. Thus, a mix of media and traditional, interpersonal communication channels have appeared to be more effective (Rogers, 1976).

Development communication approaches became more culture-specific and thwarted the dominant paradigm of seeing people as passive recipients. Participatory communication emerged as an alternative, or bottom-up, and empowering approach to influence people's perceptions and behaviour through methods and tools that were appropriately designed in local dialects for a particular community and their cultural context, aiming to reach out to literate, semi-literate as well as the illiterate population of a nation. Development communication in India employs various approaches to reach out to a diverse and multilingual population. On the one hand, it uses tools and techniques locally applied by civil society groups with very close interpersonal communication through dialogues, use of folk media and theatre. On the other, it also uses the generic, one-way communication of the government to pass on knowledge and information about various national and state-run schemes and programmes through mass media. When the aim is to cover a large population, mass media approaches are appropriate. Communication strategies employ a blend of all these methods for behaviour and attitudinal change (Figure 4.1; Table 4.2).

## 3. BEHAVIOUR CHANGE COMMUNICATION AND THE URBAN SANITATION SECTOR

Behaviour change communication (BCC) is one of the key elements of development communication with particular relevance for urban sanitation.

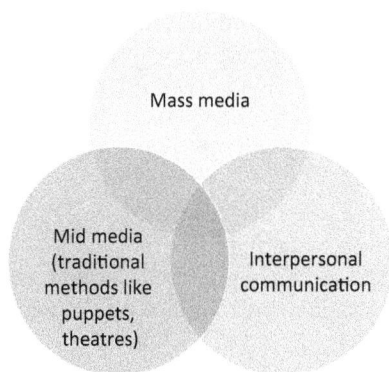

*Figure 4.1* Intermix of methods used in development communication. Source: Authors

*Table 4.2* Various approaches for development communication in India

| *Media* | | |
| --- | --- | --- |
| | Outdoor media | Hoardings, wall paintings, panels, films |
| | Mass media | TV, radio, smartphones, print (posters, illustrations), SMS |
| | Community media | Puppets, theatre, folk songs, storytelling, street plays |
| | Social media | Twitter, Facebook, WhatsApp |
| **Interpersonal communication** | | |
| *Individuals as influencers* | Celebrity (entertainment, sports) Local politicians, religious leaders Frontline workers (*Anganwadi* workers, teachers, *Mahila Aarogya Samiti* members, *Swachagrihis*, etc.) | • Focus group discussions • Dialogues • Flipbooks • Discussion cards |
| *Community groups as influencers* | *Gram* and ward *sabhas*, water and sanitation committees, slum dwellers associations, resident welfare associations, youth clubs, children's groups, self-help groups, other collectives | • Games • Pledges |

Source: Authors

Without BCC, the experiments of social innovation in this sector will not yield the expected outcomes. According to the Centre for Behaviour Change Communication, BCC positively influences knowledge, attitudes and social norms among individuals, communities and institutions. It is an interactive process of any intervention with individuals, communities and/or societies (integrated with an overall programme) to develop communication strategies to promote positive behaviours appropriate to their settings (Ngigi & Busolo, 2018). Behaviour change is now interchangeably used with social and behaviour change, which underscores the importance of behaviour change in individuals leading to collective social change for larger, social well-being.

A distinction can be made between promoting *individual change*, trying to change the behaviours in individuals that lead to social problems, promoting behaviours that lead to improved individual or social well-being, or *social change*, and attempting to mobilise public action for policy change (Coffman, 2002).

Coffman affirms that public communication campaigns use an organised set of communication activities, including all sorts of media and interpersonal communication to generate specific outcomes for a large number of individuals over a specified period. In India, popular communication campaigns through mass media include campaigns on anti-smoking, HIV/AIDS, tuberculosis, malaria, pulse polio and family planning.

In the water and sanitation sector, BCC practices have been followed for a long period, with the message that poor water and sanitation conditions impact health and the environment leading to high mortality and morbidity among the population. Safe sanitation practices include proper infrastructure, designs and technologies, but people's engagement and participation in acceptance of the technological innovations are key to achieving these safe sanitation goals. To achieve environmental, safe and healthy outcomes, laws, policies, regulations, infrastructure and service delivery mechanisms are important. At the same time, building demand for these services is equally important so that people avail them.

The strategies identified universal drivers (disgust and fear of pathogens) on which various communication campaigns were formulated.

### Participatory, intuitive-interpersonal communication approaches

Whenever participatory communication approaches are adopted, communication takes the form of dialogue to identify a problem, reflect on and articulate the problem, and analyse and solve the problem. Hence, participatory communication is a process of social change and a key element of social innovation.

**Community-Led Total Sanitation (CLTS):** Borrowing from the rural sanitation programmes and approaches, the communication strategies in urban sanitation employed various tools like mass media and interpersonal communication to transform the behaviour of the urban poor to construct toilets and use them to make the country open defecation free.

CLTS, an innovative approach in BCC, was introduced in 1999 by Kamal Kar for sanitation in rural areas in Bangladesh, India and other countries.

It proposed one universal driver – the idea of 'disgust' – as an almost universal approach to designing a set of tools. The CLTS approach in rural areas shows that after a single-day triggering event where communities are led to experience disgust at the present sanitation situation, villages achieve open defecation free (ODF) status within a month (Chambers, 2008). This approach draws on tenets of participatory research where the community is engaged in the analysis of the situation, investigating the situation and taking actions to improve the situation. Any message or new information is absorbed, processed and internalised by the community for action.

CLTS uses a participatory approach to empower local communities to stop OD and promote the building and use of latrines through community-led action instead of subsidies. The approach has shown positive results and proved to be a strong triggering mechanism for community hygiene behaviour change, especially in rural South and Southeast Asia and several African countries. In the urban context, the CLTS approach was used by Kalyani Municipality in its informal settlements, and all five slum settlements were declared ODF within six months. Later, 44 out of the 52 informal settlements in Kalyani were declared 100 percent ODF by 2007. The CLTS experience highlights the influence of subsidies, natural leaders and political will (Lüthi, 2010).

However, sanitation is much more than simply providing toilet facilities. For maintaining sanitation and hygiene-related services like solid and liquid waste management (SLWM) and faecal sludge management (FSM), an end-to-end solution is needed right from the containment of faecal waste to safe emptying, transportation, safe disposal, recycling and reuse. Non-networked sanitation systems grasped the attention of policymakers in India only from 2016 to 2017, mainly through programmes like AMRUT and SBM, as described in Chapter 1. Aligned with the shift in policy, BCC strategies too were required to shift from toilet construction to embrace the complete sanitation value.

### The dialogical process combined with mass and mid-media campaigns: community groups as influencers

To undertake a collective process of analysis and action, a dialogical process involving communication as a tool to engage the community in discussions was used in the development sector. This method of inquiry in social sciences was popularised by Paulo Freire who believed that dialogues act as a liberating mechanism and are empowering. A dialogical approach liberates people from their passivity and silence by focusing on their concrete situations and by encouraging them to verbalise their perceptions of the same. Dialogues can act as a vehicle for raising people's awareness and developing a common understanding of their present reality. The key ideas of Paulo Freire (1921–1997) are mostly explained in his well-known work, *Pedagogy of the Oppressed*. A key concept in Freire's approach is 'conscientisation', meaning how individuals and communities develop a critical understanding of their social reality through reflection and action. His work on education led to the formulation of many theories of empowerment in social sciences (Freire, 1970).

CSOs adopted participatory approaches in the communities for finding the best solutions to issues related to sanitation. The case studies discussed in this chapter illustrate how participatory communication processes led to improvement in sanitation situations in urban poor settlements.

**Centre for Urban and Regional Excellence (CURE):** CURE's work is guided by the belief that it is possible to socially innovate to meet the unmet needs of people to toilets and water taps at home and to live a life of dignity, free from poverty in an environment that is clean and pollution free. It pursues these goals through participatory processes, at the heart of which is participatory communication. It believes that community participation brings people and local governments together to discuss problems, explore options and choose best-fit solutions for their area development. It rests on the belief that people, including the poor, have local wisdom, can self-organise as networks, overcome personal differences and collaborate in reshaping their environments.

The project on improving safe and sustainable access to water and sanitation for low-income communities was implemented in the JJ[1] Colony, Sectors 8, 9 and 10 in Noida, Uttar Pradesh. This was an initiative under Corporate Social Responsibility (CSR) funded by the Dharampal Satyapal (DS) group. The project aimed to improve the quality of life of low-income communities in Noida's industrial sectors, in particular, to sustainably improve their access to safe water and toilets. CURE mobilised communities to plan and implement innovative water and sanitation solutions for in-house services and better health-seeking behaviour. By using thought-provoking methods, such as speaking to the community, the organisation effectively communicated the need for sustainable sanitation and was able to involve the community in the preparation and implementation of service improvement plans. Stimulating awareness generation methods such as nukkad natak (street play), painting slogans on walls, puppet shows and celebrating global water, sanitation and hygiene (WASH) events helped the community understand the need for safe and sustainable sanitation practices.

**Nidan:** Nidan institutes networks and committees in slum communities and leverages its existing relationships with workers' groups within informal settlements in Patna to extend its services to urban sanitation – a need felt within those communities. With enlightened group members acting as 'sanitation champions', Nidan mobilises households around sanitation, with continuous behaviour change messaging playing a key role. Nidan uses group meetings, informal settlement education centres and schools to spread sanitation and hygiene awareness. At the core of Nidan's innovation is the coming together of the infrastructure of toilet construction for this section of the community with investment in behaviour modification and its proactive engagement as a bridge between the community and the sanitation service providers. Both technical solutions and access to services are combined in this innovative approach with behaviour change as an intended outcome.

Another key approach adopted by Nidan as part of its innovations in urban sanitation is multisectoral. Using communication strategies, it actively engages with the government and liaises and works to break through various developmental silos so that sanitation is seen as an integrated city-wide agenda. It recognises that even though sanitation may appear to be a municipality or urban ministry issue, it is closely engaged in health, social work, education and livelihood. This holistic approach is translated in many of its sanitation projects, such as sanitation campaigns in schools and *Anganwadis*.

While adults are important stakeholders targeted by the BCC campaigns in sanitation, children are another stakeholder group who are targeted by CSOs. Behaviour change begins at home and through a process that engages family members. Children who learn to practice health and hygiene (like hand washing and toilet use) in schools become key messengers and influencers in the family to communicate about health and hygiene. UNICEF, WaterAid and many CSOs engaged with these development partners, including Gramalaya, have worked with children and youth to create a wider impact on their home and their community.

**Development Alternatives (DA):** DA started its dedicated urban sanitation work in the last decade with a small initiative to build the capacities of masons to construct toilets and facilitate technological innovations related to prefabricated toilets with recyclable materials. Apart from technologically innovative toilet solutions and scattered capacity-building initiatives, the lion's share of the major urban sanitation works of DA to date revolves around BCC. Like in all other aspects of its work, DA's innovations in urban sanitation are guided by its organisational values of social equity and environmental equality.

Although the primary focus of the CLEAN India programme was not urban sanitation, WASH initiatives to improve associated facilities for urban dwellers have been an area of attention of the DA group. Through this initiative, the group has designed a water filter package besides a complete sanitation package consisting of toilets, soak pits and drainage systems. Launched by CLEAN India, a flagship programme of DA, 'The City I Want' campaign is a youth-led social media initiative aimed at improving the current environmental scenario of cities in India. To set the base of the campaign, an online survey has been undertaken to understand the concerns of the youth regarding emerging environmental challenges. As part of the campaign, the urban youth are envisaged to be encouraged to identify and articulate pressing urban issues, propose solutions and commit to taking actions for a better tomorrow.

The idea behind this unique initiative involving young children was to project the future citizens as spearheads of change and influence all other stakeholders in a structured framework with the flexibility to address local needs. DA has followed the '4 As Approach' to manage the entire CLEAN initiative – assessment, awareness, action and advocacy. Such an approach can be elaborated as follows: Systematic **assessment** of environmental quality, including sanitation, of major cities and towns by a network of schools underpinned by non-governmental organisation (NGO) partners and validated by the government, followed by large-scale **awareness** led by school students to influence communities and initiate **action** demonstrating good practices and ultimately resulting in **advocacy** for informed policy change. Although the programme was initially started to cover urban areas, it has spread to peri-urban areas as well.

### *Immersion and formative research to design and implement mass media campaigns rooted in cultural context*

Fear of diseases and avoidance of pathogens are universal across cultures, with all societies demonstrating individual- and group-level hygiene behaviours. In the sanitation sector, the communication strategies related to hand washing, construction of toilets, abatement of OD practices and wastewater management have largely banked upon the universal driver of fear (of pathogens) and disgust. To some extent, this approach was successful in driving behaviour change. It usually works when most of the culture recognises some objects as universally impure, such as human faeces and pathogens.

> In order for behaviour to change, people must feel personally vulnerable to a health threat, view the possible consequences as severe, and see that taking action is likely to either prevent or reduce the risk at an acceptable cost with few barriers. In addition, a person must feel competent (have self-efficacy) to execute and maintain the new behaviour. Some trigger, either internal ... or external ... is required to ensure actual behaviour ensues.
>
> (Nisbet & Gick, 2008)

The health belief model (HBM) (Hochbaum, 1958; Rosenstock, 1966; Becker, 1974; Sharma & Romas, 2012) is a cognitive model, which posits that behaviour is determined by several beliefs about threats to an individual's well-being and the effectiveness and outcomes of particular actions or behaviours. Some constructions of the model feature the concept of self-efficacy (Bandura, 1997), alongside these beliefs about actions. These beliefs are further supplemented by additional stimuli referred to as 'cues to action', which trigger the actual adoption of behaviour. **Perceived threat** is at the core of the HBM as it is linked to a person's 'readiness' to take action. It consists of two sets of beliefs about an individual's **perceived**

**susceptibility or vulnerability** to a particular threat and the seriousness of the expected consequences that may result from it. The **perceived benefits** associated with a behaviour, which is its likely effectiveness in reducing the threat, are weighed against the perceived costs of any negative consequences that may result from it (**perceived barriers**) to establish the overall extent to which a behaviour is beneficial. The individual's perceived capacity to adopt the behaviour (their **self-efficacy**) is a further key component of the model. Finally, the HBM identifies two types of 'cue to action' – internal and external. These cues affect the perception of threats and can trigger or maintain behaviour.

### Box 4.1 Malasur Campaign – Demon of Defeca

BBC Media Action (BBC MA), in partnership with the state-level technical support units (TSUs) and with funding from the Bill and Melinda Gates Foundation (BMGF), designed an evidence-based, insight-driven Social and Behaviour Change Communication (SBCC) intervention to heighten risk perception around FSSM. BBC MA conducted formative research (qualitative exploration and quantitative survey) at Narsapur (Telangana), Trichy (Tamil Nadu) and Berhampur (Odisha) among 1,740 households to assess the barriers, triggers, attitudes and current practices towards FSSM. The research showed apathy towards properly constructed onsite sanitation systems, timely desludging of septic tanks and unsafe disposal of faecal waste in an open environment. Based on the formative research, the communication objectives were to increase awareness, heighten risk perception and build a sense of urgency. The basic tenet for the campaign was to raise the profile of FSM by positioning faecal sludge as a clear and present danger to households, if ignored. The team worked through an idea that was insight-driven, user-centric, media-agnostic and disruptive. The team focused on using Indian mythology and the traditional tales of good and evil, of gods and demons. Consequently, Malasur – the demon of defeca – was conceptualised. Malasur is a visual personification of faecal sludge. Malasur is this unseen demon who lives under your feet, bubbling away, biding its time, waiting until that opportune moment when it can erupt into a backflow or an overflow. Malasur is a threat to your water unless you build the right kind of septic tank, do regular desludging and keep an eye on where your faecal sludge is being dumped. A 360-degree campaign was developed using film, radio, outdoor, GIFs, outreach material and a comprehensive toolkit to enable stakeholders (government and non-government) to implement the campaign across different geographies and platforms. The Malasur campaign and toolkit (in 11 languages to help implement the campaign) were unveiled by the Minister of State, Ministry of Housing and Urban Affairs, on 5 June 2020 – the World Environment Day – marking FSSM as a national priority and establishing Malasur as the national campaign on FSSM. The toolkit contains all Malasur campaign collaterals or outputs in ready-to-print, open files across various platforms. These are outputs on outdoor media (hoardings, wall paintings), in-transit media (cesspool truck, auto rickshaw/van), mid-media (miking, street play) and audio-visuals (cinema slides, animation films, GIFs). These have been developed in 11 languages to cater to the language diversity in India. The campaign has been rolled out across Warangal (Telangana), Rajam (Andhra Pradesh), 114 urban local bodies in Odisha and also in Madhya Pradesh and Uttar Pradesh. In the first two weeks after its launch on social media, the film earned 525,000 impressions on Twitter and was watched more than 300,000 times. The Malasur campaign has been piloted, pre-tested and evaluated, providing valuable learning on how to design communication strategies and solutions around FSSM behaviours (NFSSM Alliance & NITI Aayog, 2021).

**Centre for Policy Research (CPR):** Project Nirmal was implemented by the Centre for Policy Research (CPR) and Practical Action (PA) in Angul and Dhenkanal (Odisha) during 2015–2020 to demonstrate FSM pilots with the support of BMGF and Arghyam. The project started (2015) when there was not much awareness among government stakeholders and small-town communities on non-networked sanitation systems. The attitude and behaviours related to safe practices of proper containment, emptying, transportation and disposal of faecal sludge (FS) were virtually absent. Before developing a BCC plan and strategy, the project undertook formative research in the informal settlements of both towns and found that the residents were largely aware about open defecation practices and that open disposal of faeces is harmful as their own traditional cultures considered human excreta as defiling. Ethnographic research on culture and sanitation in these towns also showed that people were not averse to building toilets despite space constraints; but in the absence of any awareness of the construction of properly designed toilets and onsite sanitation systems (OSS), lack of finances, absence of any mechanical processes for emptying and disposal of faecal sludge, the community faced tremendous challenges.

So, while the universal driver of disgust was present in the absence of any other arrangements, communities were forced to practice OD or have unsanitary OSS. The practice of manual emptying was rampant, and pollution of land and water owing to indiscriminate disposal of waste was also known. The project found that building awareness on toilet construction to check OD would not have led to any change if technical know-how, financing and proper FSM were not in place. The campaign was designed to not only focus on building toilets to end OD but to get the right OSS built and strengthen FSM. Since the project aimed at providing sustainable FSM services, the BCC was designed to focus on why cities of small sizes need FSM, what are the current practices, how they can be supported in this initiative, and how communities can draw out an action plan to spread awareness in informal settlements on the complete value chain of FSM, which included safe containment, safe emptying, safe transportation and safe disposal. The campaign also underscored the importance of non-hazardous cleaning and eradicating manual emptying processes that were hazardous for sanitary workers. The formative research also identified youth groups, elected representatives and women as champions in the community who could lead the campaign by involving other community members.

Another important lesson from this case was that BCC is an evolving and dynamic process. Depending on the stages of interventions of any project or programme, the focus of BCC also desires a shift. In the initial phases of environment building through community discussions, proper design of toilets with onsite sanitation systems and use of toilets was the focus, which evolved to include messages on the complete value chain of FSM, the role of each stakeholder, prevention of manual scavenging, regular desludging of onsite sanitation systems, safe transportation and disposal. When the FS treatment plant was built, the BCC campaigns focused on the awareness of safe emptying and disposal. Project partners circulated information to the community in informal settlements with call centre numbers and the fee for desludging to enable the community to access services.

Community-level groups of informal settlement dwellers, ward members, self-help group members, Mahila Aarogya Samiti members, youth groups and swachhagrahis were forerunners in the campaign. The BCC campaigns were a mix of interpersonal and mass media (posters, hoarding, wall painting, miking through vans, etc.). These campaigns were empowering for the citizens as they began to demand accountability from the government on quicker desludging services. Once the voices from the community become stronger, improvement in water and solid waste management in urban poor locations was also witnessed. The monitoring data of desludging requests by urban households doubled in three months due to increased BCC campaigns in both towns.

**Participatory Research in Asia (PRIA):** The work of PRIA highlights the importance of communication among residents of informal settlements for social innovations in urban sanitation to be successful. Through its Engaged Citizens Responsive City (ECRC) initiatives in three Indian cities (Ajmer, Jhansi and Muzaffarpur), PRIA emphasised collective behaviour change in low-income communities living in the informal settlements of these cities. PRIA facilitated the formation of Settlement Improvement Committees with leadership from young women and men to act as change agents within the committee. These young women and men from the community analysed the sanitation situation in each settlement holistically through participatory settlement enumeration (PSE) and participatory urban appraisal (PUA) tools and shared the findings with fellow community members. The identified service gaps and reasons thereof were discussed with the entire community for preparing community action plans. The horizontal communication between the residents of informal settlements deepened the sense of agency to promote healthy sanitary practices in the community. PRIA provided critical information about service provisions under various public sanitation programmes and how the community could benefit from such programmes, particularly in accessing subsidised individual household toilets (IHHTs) and community/public toilets (CT/PT) towards the eradication of OD practices. This facilitated increased demands for both IHHTs and CT/PTs.

This horizontal communication also catalysed increased interactions among the urban local body (ULB) officials, local councillors and settlement improvement committee (SIC) leadership to jointly plan for accessing better sanitation services in the settlements, including regular cleaning of public spaces, garbage collection and utilisation of newly constructed IHHTs and CT/PTs. The initial success provided momentum to community-led information and education campaigns with critical support from the ULBs. The community members who were previously either ignorant or indifferent to various government BCC campaigns began to not only take an active interest but also led various campaigns. Several youth leaders from the SICs led Swachh Survekshan (a performance ranking exercise for cities vis-à-vis sanitation led by the GOI) and ban single-use plastic, disaggregation of household waste, reduce open defecation and urination and improve the overall environment in the settlements.

The ECRC experience of PRIA emphasised that top-down development communication towards behaviour change needs to be complemented with local organising and preparing change agents within the community for better impact. The intended message from the top-down communication must be demystified and internalised by the community for facilitating actual behaviour change in the community. The community change agents are best placed to facilitate this collective internalisation. Also, while behaviour change at the individual level is critical, this can be accelerated by promoting a collective critical consciousness. The role of an intermediary agency, such as PRIA in this case, has been to access information from external institutions and disseminate them in a simplified fashion to the community members to analyse, internalise and act upon without imposing a forced behaviour change. The increased interactions between the resident low-income community of the informal settlements and the ULB officials and elected councillors also facilitated a change in the behaviour of the latter. Having been exposed to the realities of informal settlement dwellers, many ULB officials and councillors became much more sensitive and responsive to the plight of these deprived communities. They sincerely tried to address major service gaps in the settlements.

Print materials in form of posters and graphic illustrations are used to reduce the complexities of technical sanitation issues and make them more understandable. A comic book, *A Sludge Story*, published by Consortium for Decentralised Wastewater Treatment Systems (DEWATS) dissemination (CDD), captures a story of sludge and wastewater treatment in a lucid manner. The protagonist of *A Sludge Story*, Buland Babu, is a common man who wishes nothing but the best for his city. Buland Babu educates as well as raises awareness about the need for human waste treatment that does not come at a cost to the environment.

People's behaviour is influenced by personal as well as environmental and social factors so the BCC strategies need to employ learning from the experiences of others who are part of the same ecosystem. Social cognitive theory (SCT), the cognitive formulation of social learning theory, best articulated by Bandura, explains human behaviour in terms of a three-way, dynamic, reciprocal model wherein personal factors, environmental influences and behaviour continually interact. This is often known as *reciprocal determinism* (that a person can be both an agent for change and a responder to change).

Environmental factors represent situational influences and the environment in which behaviour is performed, while personal factors include instincts, drives, traits and other individual motivational forces. Several constructs underlie the process of human learning and behaviour change.

A basic premise of SCT is that people learn not only through their own experiences but also by observing the actions of others and the results of those actions. Therefore, peer learning and pilot interventions enable people to learn from others' experiences. In SBM, to motivate the urban poor households to construct toilets with proper onsite sanitation systems, the experience of other community members who had built affordable, onsite sanitation systems was a catalyst for effecting behaviour change in the community through peer learning. Many innovative practices and strategies employed by cities on FSSM were transmitted to other cities and states through films and videos.

## 4. CONCLUSION

Strategic communication on urban sanitation is key to achieving SDG 6 on safe sanitation. With increasing focus on FSSM in the country, communication campaigns are pivotal in sustaining the technological innovations and investments made by the government.

Development communication has gained recognition in India's development practices, and urban sanitation is no exception. Major national programmes and schemes on water and sanitation in India place greater importance on behaviour change, implying that communication approaches can change the behaviour of citizens and adopt new practices for larger individuals and the public good. Any technological innovations and infrastructure gains on sanitation can be put to effective use when they can become sustainable with strategic communication approaches.

Development communication approaches have evolved from being top-down to becoming more participative. Various social innovations in communication strategies by CSOs, as illustrated in this chapter, have facilitated a shift of behaviour to impact health and environmental outcomes coupled with enabling communities to meet their basic needs.

As demonstrated through case studies, awareness generation and enhanced knowledge and information also led to greater accountability and improved service delivery due to greater demand by the community. Greater knowledge of the use of toilets and improved health of onsite sanitation systems created demand on ULBs to provide quick and efficient services of timely desludging of onsite sanitation systems, creating decentralised systems for FSM.

Development communication, as we have observed in this chapter through various case studies, employs a mix of methods – from being top-down to engaging participatory tools for people to analyse their existing situation and find out the best possible alternative to change for a better outcome to meet unmet needs. Social innovations around communication strategies stem from participatory research, strongly anchored in valuing indigenous knowledge and cultural relativism. CSOs have played a key role in raising the critical consciousness of communities to change their behaviour and attitudes to embrace transformation. While the role of CSOs has been critical in catalysing behaviour changes through social innovations, the government's role in diffusing the innovations through policy changes is also critical. Small-scale interventions by CSOs in some geographies can be adopted at a large scale with some context-specific adaptations, as illustrated by the case studies in this chapter, for changes at the individual, institutional and societal levels to meet the unmet needs of urban sanitation.

A key aim of the behaviour change explored in this chapter is to raise a new public consciousness around sanitation work and social attitudes towards those who undertake this critical function. The next chapter, 'Sanitation Work and Workers: Prioritising Issues of Rights, Dignity and Safety', foregrounds social innovations around the rights and dignity of sanitation workers.

## Note

1 JJ: *Jhuggi Jhopri*, meaning hutments or informal housing or settlements.

# 5 Sanitation Work and Workers
## Prioritising Issues of Rights, Dignity and Safety

## 1. INTRODUCTION

This chapter analyses the work of a host of civil society innovations, which have contributed to raising a new public consciousness around sanitation work, enabled access to the rights and dignity of sanitation workers and reduced the drudgery of sanitation work. It traces the evolution of laws, policies and programmes directed at ameliorating the dismal condition of sanitation workers, particularly manual scavengers, while pointing to the problem of lackadaisical implementation and lack of accountability of public institutions.

On the global front, SDG 8 calls for 'full and productive employment and decent work for all women and men' and to 'protect labour rights and promote safe and secure working environments for all workers, including migrant workers, particularly women migrants, and those in precarious employment'. The International Labour Organization (ILO) (2014), as per its definitions of 'decent work', gives manual scavengers a legal identity under the law as workers, enabling them to exercise rights. ILO further distinguishes three forms of manual scavenging: (i) removal of human excrement from public streets and dry latrines, (ii) cleaning of septic tanks and (iii) cleaning of gutters and sewers.

There are almost five million sanitation workers nationally, half of whom are women (PRIA, 2019). National surveys to identify manual scavengers in the country have been distorted by blatant disrespect and suspicion of the community, accentuated further by the state authorities' denial of the situation and disowning responsibility for eradicating manual scavenging.

Not only is the very nature of sanitation work hazardous, but the working conditions of sanitation workers in India are rendered even more precarious by the occupation's inescapable association with the caste system. This links sanitation as the sole concern of the scheduled castes, particularly the Valmiki community. Adding another layer of complexity is the gender fault line with women sanitation workers living and working under the double burden of labour (wage earners as well as caregivers in the household).

DOI: 10.4324/9781003197102-5

The Protection of Civil Rights Act, 1955, The Employment of Manual Scavengers and Construction of Dry Latrines (Prohibition) (EMSCDLP) Act, 1993, and Prohibition of Employment as Manual Scavengers and their Employment (PEMSR) Act, 2013, by the Ministry of Social Justice and Empowerment as well as schemes and programmes offered by public commissions and corporations such as the National Commission for Safai Karmacharis (NCSK), National Safai Karamchari Financial Development Corporation (NSKFDC) and SBM address the socio-economic and working rights of sanitation workers. Yet, there continue to exist multilayered systemic gaps that keep sanitation workers socio-economically marginalised and deprived.

The examples of various development organisations – like the Safai Karamchari Andolan (SKA) and Jan Sahas – have underscored efforts to mobilise sanitation workers and public opinion against manual scavenging. The work of Participatory Research in Asia (PRIA) highlights the gender dimension of sanitation work, while that of Centre for Policy Research (CPR) uses research from equity and inclusive lenses to connect policymakers and organisations of sanitation workers by highlighting the precarious working conditions of the workers and their lack of accessibility to various government programmes and schemes.

The problems central to the safety and dignity of sanitation work have remained deeply entrenched for many years. Though focused efforts and investments have been made to analyse the issue and find solutions through work mechanisation and legislative reforms, the concerns still loom large in various forms. Vulnerabilities of caste-related sanitation work have persisted for a long time and seem to have become deeply ingrained in the work itself. This chapter deliberates and discusses sanitation work-related vulnerabilities and how they manifest in the subjects of safety, dignity and rights of the sanitation workers.

## 2. HISTORICAL LANDSCAPE OF RIGHTS AND ENTITLEMENTS OF SANITATION WORKERS

The relationship between caste and manual scavenging is not simple. Literature extensively describes how caste plays a role in discrimination or politics, such as Teltumbde (2010 and 2014) who highlighted how caste has been politicised in India to the detriment of manual scavengers. There are some studies dedicated to the discussion on the caste of manual scavengers. One of the studies linking caste and manual scavenging is by Pradhan (1938), who discussed that 80 percent of the 'depressed classes' working in Bombay city (the Marathi-speaking Mahars and the Gujarati-speaking Meghwals and Bhangis) were employed in manual scavenging. The study attempted to present how religious conversion did not alter the economic condition of the 'depressed classes' and formed a vicious circle for many to do manual scavenging work. There are other studies on caste and manual scavengers, which date back to the colonial era, with one of the earliest studies by Prashad (1995) dedicated to the 'sweeper' castes (Mehtars, Chuhras and Balmikis), arguing how the colonial government has perpetuated scavenging. This finding was further corroborated by Chaplin (1999), who put forth the argument that because of the weak sanitation movement and weak local governments in Indian cities, the informal sanitation workers are subservient to middle-class interests.

Emancipation of manual scavengers is a significant focus of the literature on Dalit studies in general and manual scavenging in particular. One noteworthy example is that of Prashad (1995) wherein he traces the history of the emancipation of untouchables between 1920 and 1950, suppressing and ignoring the political potential of sweepers' strikes and associations through the adoption of workers' rights and Gandhian (rights-based spiritual solution) approaches to the freedom struggle. In short, these approaches not only lowered the voice of untouchables for economic demands but also reduced their cry for humanity to a question of the provision of decent implements and showers.

In another study, D'Sourza (2016) traces the impact of urbanisation on manual scavenging in Ahmedabad. The study found that among the migrants from rural to urban areas, the lower castes are stopped from moving up the occupation ladder.

> Over three generations one observes that the members of the marginal castes from rural areas who were predominantly agricultural labourers in the rural economy are assimilated into the urban labour market as scavengers first largely in the organised sector in local bodies and then in the informal sector.
>
> (Ibid.)

The unsafe and undignified practice of sanitation work, including manually cleaning excrement from private and public dry toilets and open drains, persists in India to a large extent. Within the sanitation workspace, there is a hierarchy between sweeper communities and manual scavengers Chaplin 2011). Owing to the notion of dignity and purity, sweepers feel superior to manual scavengers as they do not carry human excreta and are paid a pension. The sanitation workspace highlights the gender divide that exists in the scavenging work wherein women scavenge private households because they are not strong enough for mechanised garbage collection or sewer cleaning (ibid.). Consistent with a centuries-old feudal custom, most of the work of 'manual scavengers' is undertaken by women and low-caste communities who collect human waste on a daily basis, load it into cane baskets or metal troughs and carry it away on their heads for disposal at the outskirts of the settlement.

For decades the sanitation workspace has reported direct, cultural and structural violence suffered by sanitation workers, particularly manual scavengers (Shahid, 2015). Violence has been felt at two levels – social violence of caste discrimination as well as the threat of physical violence as a result of caste discrimination and job conditions. Furthermore, the cultural context around caste attenuates and justifies the structural violence against manual scavengers (ibid.). Ramaiah (2011) articulates the considerably increasing incidences of criminal acts against Dalits and scheduled castes from 1981 to 1999.

Manual scavenging has existed in India since the pre-independence era, despite the government's legislative and policy efforts in the sanitation space. Several committees or task forces have been constituted to inform government policies and programmes ensuring safety and dignity in the sanitation space. The earliest Barve Committee (The Scavengers' Living Conditions Enquiry Committee 1949–1952) led to a scheme for the supply of wheel-barrows and improved implements to scavengers to eliminate the practice of 'head loading' where night soil was carried on the heads of manual scavengers for disposal. The Kalelkar Commission Report (Backward Classes Commission, 1953–1955) highlighted the 'sub-human' conditions under which manual scavengers worked, including carrying night soil on their heads using leaky receptacles and living in segregated communities. This was followed by a review of sweepers and scavengers' inhumane working conditions by the Central Advisory Board for Harijan Welfare, constituted under the Malkani Committee (or the Scavenging Conditions Enquiry Committee), 1958–1960.

To try and dignify the sanitation space, the Committee on Customary Rights to Scavengers in 1969 was formed to examine the absence of municipal sanitation services and customary relationships developed between scavengers and households where latrines were cleaned by the former. In 1966, the Gadkar Committee's report called for legislation to regulate service conditions and set up an inspectorate, which was reiterated later by the Pandya Committee. Despite government efforts, the focus remained on the conversion of dry latrines over complete rehabilitation (Basu, 1991). Overall, the committees recommended improvements in the living and working conditions of scavengers, which included technological interventions to improve their working conditions through systematic conversion of dry latrines into pour-flush latrines.

While the committees articulated the issue of manual scavenging to be resolved through technological solutions, the focus rested on research and policy-oriented efforts, which dwelt on the subjects of sanitation infrastructure, mechanisation of work and the dehumanising aspect of the oppressed practice. Though the committees and working groups took cognizance of eradicating manual scavenging, the GOI passed two acts in 1993 and 2013, offering technical and social solutions to end manual scavenging. The former (1993) focused on eliminating dry and insanitary latrines, while the latter (2013) intensified efforts on the rehabilitation of manual scavengers. A more recent report of the sub-group on Safai Karamcharis (2007) prepared for the 11th Five-Year Plan, identified manual scavengers, sewer workers and sanitation workers as the most vulnerable. The sub-group called for the total eradication of manual scavenging by implementing labour laws and adequate workplace safety.

In 2013, The Employment of Manual Scavengers and Construction of Dry Latrines (Prohibition) Act, 1993, was amended to include all those who worked without adequate physical safety protection and safety gear, through direct human contact to manually clean human faecal waste. The resulting legislation, Prohibition of Employment as Manual Scavengers and their Rehabilitation Act, 2013, was expected to be a game-changer. The 2013 law details the need for and process of rehabilitation of identified manual scavengers. Even before the law was passed, the Ministry of Social Justice and Empowerment in 2007 introduced the Self-Employment Scheme for Rehabilitation of Manual Scavengers (SRMS) to rehabilitate manual scavengers and their dependents in a time-bound manner by March 2009. The SRMS scheme is aimed at cash assistance, capital and interest subsidy for enterprises, skill training and loans for identified manual scavengers.

---

**Box 5.1 Self-Employment Scheme for Rehabilitation of Manual Scavengers (SRMS)**

SRMS is a centrally sponsored scheme introduced by the Ministry of Social Justice and Empowerment in 2007. It aims to rehabilitate manual scavengers and their dependents in alternative occupations. It provides one-time cash assistance of Rs 40,000 to either the identified manual scavenger or a family member. A loan of up to Rs 10 lakh is admissible under the scheme for self-employment projects. An additional Rs 5 lakh is admissible in case the identified beneficiary takes up sanitation-related projects involving vacuum loaders, suction machine vehicles and garbage disposal vehicles. It also includes the provision of course training for two years with a monthly stipend of Rs 3,000. The guidelines recognise these sanitation-related projects as 'extremely relevant for the target group'. This scheme is implemented by the National Safai Karmacharis Finance and Development Corporation.

*Source*: NSKFDC (n.d.)

---

While these policies, programmes and rehabilitation schemes have not been able to completely translate their objectives, sanitation workers have not yet been able to fully cognise their rights and entitlements. Thus, as witnessed in the earlier **campaigns and rights-oriented** initiatives of organisations, they have yielded towards reinforcing the rights and entitlements of sanitation workers, further protecting them from the threats of violence and expulsion from their community.

## 3. MISSING LINKS IN SAFE AND DIGNIFIED SANITATION WORK

Scholars have attempted to understand manual scavenging as a typology of sanitation-based activities and choices rather than the traditional focus of just caste-based social injustice faced by manual scavengers. For example, a study by Dak (2007) to assess the impact of the National Scheme of Liberation and Rehabilitation of Scavengers (NSLRS) in Rajasthan found that until dry latrines were converted into pour-flush latrines, scavenging would remain a problem. It concluded that 'the condition of the scavenging population is determined mainly by the quality of toilets and availability of flush arrangements' (ibid.). Another report on the National Urban Sanitation policy called for the manual cleaning of septic tanks to be recognised as manual scavenging (Rohilla & Trivedi, 2011).

Though the sanitation space is embedded in the legal framework, policies and working committees for legislative and rehabilitative measures, the issue of correct estimation of manual scavengers in the country persists. There have been seven national surveys in the past 26 years to identify manual scavengers in the country. A survey conducted in 1992 identified 5.88 lakh manual scavengers, while another study by the Ministry of Social Justice and Empowerment (2002–2003) recognised 6.76 lakh manual scavengers in India (The Wire, 2018). There was an upward revision of the numbers to the tune of nearly 8 lakh (7,70,338) manual scavengers and even more till the Census 2011 was conducted. It was very ironic to see a decline in numbers to a few thousand, just 54,300 in a 2018 nationwide survey (across 18 states), commissioned after the publishing of The Prohibition of Employment as Manual Scavengers and their Rehabilitation Act (ibid.).

The statistics are further skewed in the context of the rehabilitation of manual scavengers under SRMS. As per the Ministry of Social Justice and Empowerment, only 1.18 lakh of the 3.42 lakh manual scavengers and their dependents in 18 states/UTs were identified for SRMS; and only 78,941 manual scavengers have claimed assistance of loans at subsidised interest rates and credit-linked capital subsidy for self-employment (The Wire, 2018).

The ministry claims to have assisted 78,941 manual scavengers out of 1.18 lakh scavengers, with loans at subsidised interest rates and credit-linked capital subsidy for self-employment. There has been no follow-up action since then, nor any rehabilitation of the remaining 2.6 lakh manual scavengers who were identified and then left high and dry. Government data records that after the new legislation was passed in 2013, claims of only 12,771 manual scavengers received the one-time cash assistance and only 4,587 received skill development training (The Wire, 2018).

The disparity in the surveys depicts a different story with the designing process and blatant disrespect and suspicion of the community marring the outlined mandate. This has been furthered by the state and district authorities' denial of the situation and more so by disowning the responsibility of eradicating manual scavenging.

Sanitation is often seen as the social good promoting health and hygiene, as well as the propagator of unsafe and undignified work for sanitation workers. Besides being a perpetrator of hard and unprotected labour, sanitation perniciously marks the absence of any safety gear leading to reports of injuries such as burns, choking and breathlessness. Adequate monetary compensation, reskilling and entrepreneurship support are some of the missing elements of the sanitation workspace across wide categories of sanitation workers.

The categories of sanitation workers are broadly defined across the levels of engagement, ranging from permanent government employees, daily wage workers with government agencies and local bodies, subcontractors or staff of private sector agencies or NGOs, or informal workers and entrepreneurs. Their job is characterised by different shades of formality and non-formality, which also determine the kinds of benefits from the government schemes they can access. A detailed presentation of the categories of sanitation workers on the levels of vulnerability and engagement is visualised in Figure 5.1, based on the study conducted by the Centre for Policy Research (Dasgupta et al., 2020).

However, because policies fail to be adequately implemented, sanitation workers stay in denial of their rights and persistently face intense social pressure and violence. Amid all the technological and social efforts by varied development organisations (see Table 5.1), what persist are the issues of safety and dignity, as well as the cycle of caste oppression and poverty dehumanisation, which exemplify the scope of partnership models of sanitation workers deliberating the following: (a) recognising the sanitation workers as workers and as human beings who have been historically marginalised; (b) promoting working conditions and social protection that match their recognition as workers and (c) breaking the vicious cycle of caste through the lens of oppression, dehumanisation and poverty.

## 4. INTERVENTIONS BY CSOs TO UPHELD RIGHTS AND DIGNITY OF SANITATION WORKERS

In the following sections, examples of relevant work have been broadly discussed under two categories: (a) campaigns and rights-oriented work and (b) policy and research-oriented work.

### Campaigns and rights-oriented work

Drawing tenets from social change theories, mobilisation and organisation building of oppressed and marginalised through the awakening of their

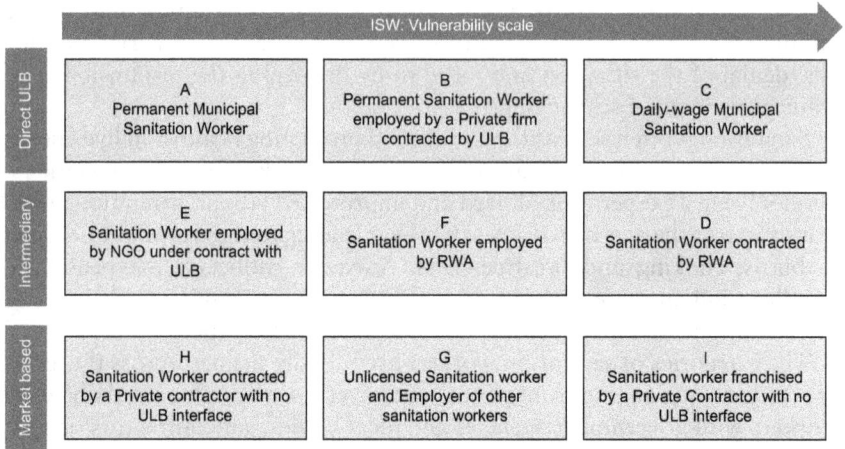

*Figure 5.1* Sanitation workers' categories. Source: Adapted from Dasgupta et al., 2020

consciousness to demand their rights remained central to many social innovations carried out by civil society organisations.

**Safai Karamchari Andolan:** SKA has championed the concerns of manual scavengers and is committed towards the abolition of the dehumanising practice of manual scavenging and dignified rehabilitation for those who have undertaken this work of physically removing untreated human excreta using the most basic tools.

Since 1982, SKA has been raising its voice against this discrimination and has organised, mobilised and campaigned against this atrocity for the discontinuation of dry latrines, and its link with the dehumanising occupation of scavenging. It is widely seen as a movement that aims to completely eradicate manual scavenging from India. The movement began with the efforts of the youth from the community, led by Bezwada Wilson. Mr Wilson, a national convener of the SKA and recipient of the Ramon Magsaysay Award 2016 for his work on manual scavengers, hailed from the same Dalit community and 'started responding to reality' with the idea of augmenting dignity, self-respect and equality for *safai karmacharis*. The centenary celebration of Dr BR Ambedkar during 1990 opened a window for Mr Wilson to learn more about the teachings of Dr Ambedkar and draw on these learnings on the dynamics of caste and social class, which were used to articulate the core values of the organisation.

Mr Bezwada Wilson initiated a cycle yatra in Kolar region and introduced the ideas of BR Ambedkar – to educate, agitate and organise the manual scavenging eradication movement. Armed with this, country-wide protests were organised at District Magistrate offices, and petitions were submitted to the collector to end the practice of manual scavenging. When the government did not act on their pleas, the women from the community

*Table 5.1* Approach adopted by different organisations

| Organisations | Campaigns and rights-oriented work | Research and policy-oriented work |
|---|---|---|
| Safai Karamchari Andolan | • Mass movement<br>• Networking with like-minded organisations | |
| Jan Sahas | • Rastriya Garima Abhiyan, a national-level campaign<br>• Networking with partner organisations | |
| Chintan | • Campaigns<br>• Collectivisation of the informal workers | |
| Centre for Policy Research | | • Effectiveness of SRMS scheme – Punjab<br>• Invisible sanitation workers' study |
| Participatory Research in Asia | | • Bodies of Accumulation – A Study on Women Sanitation Workers<br>• Lived Realities of Women Sanitation Workers in India – Study across Three Cities in India |
| Urban Management Centre | | • Technical assistance through technical support units for Garima Scheme<br>• Handbook – Training of sanitation workers on PPEs<br>• Ensuring Safety of Sanitation Workers – A Ready Reckoner for Urban Local Bodies |
| Water Aid – Centre for Equity Studies | | • Research studies on manual scavenging |
| SWaCH | | • Formation of a waste collectors' cooperative |

*Source*: Authors

– who were the primary victims of this practice – lead a movement across the country to demolish dry latrines. This is how SKA came into being in 1993.

In 1993, the parliament passed The Employment of Manual Scavengers and Construction of Dry Latrines (Prohibition) Act, 1993, with imprisonment for up to one year and/or a fine of Rs 2,000. This law never led to convictions in the last couple of decades, while the government made repeated promises to eliminate this heinous practice. Following that, in 2003, SKA filed a Public Interest Litigation (PIL) in the Supreme Court – asking it to ensure the eradication of dry latrines and to recognise that manual scavenging violated the fundamental rights of the people doing such work. A total denial from the state governments about the existence of manual scavenging was followed by partial admission when SKA produced photographic evidence and, finally, compliance to some extent.

In 2007, with the solidarity and support of civil society groups and public leaders, SKA launched the Action 2010 campaign to end manual scavenging by December 2010. When nothing seemed to be making a difference, SKA started the historic 'Samajik Parivartan Yatra' in October 2010. This bus *yatra*, which was the first of its kind, journeyed the entire country with many women and men, who had left manual scavenging, leading it. It ended with a massive public meeting in Delhi.

In addition, SKA submitted memorandums to the President, Prime Minister, Ministries, statutory bodies and the National Advisory Council (NAC) for the implementation of the 1993 Act and a rehabilitation package. The NAC passed a resolution on 23 October 2010 to end manual scavenging by 31 March 2012. It was after the Yatra, the then Minister of Social Justice and Empowerment called SKA for a discussion. It was in that meeting SKA shared the nationwide data collected during the *yatra* and presented skewed government statistics on the number of registered and rehabilitated manual scavengers.

Following the meeting, the Ministry of Social Justice and Empowerment convened the national consultation on 24 and 25 January 2011, which resulted in the setting up of four task forces – to review the act, conduct a national survey and revise the rehabilitation package and sanitation solutions. The President of India in her speech to the parliament at the start of the budget session in March 2012 announced the draft of a new bill for the prohibition of manual scavenging. The GOI passed the new 'Prohibition of Employment as Manual Scavengers and Their Rehabilitation Act' in September 2013 and issued the government notification in December 2013.

Further, after 12 long years, the Supreme Court passed its judgment order on 27 March 2014 on the writ petition (civil) number 583 of 2003, SKA & Others versus Union of India & Ors., directing all the state governments and the Union Territories to (i) fully implement and take appropriate action for non-implementation as well as violation of the provisions contained in the 2013 Act, (ii) prevent deaths in sewer holes and septic tanks and make the manual cleaning of sewers and septic tanks a crime even in emergency situations and (iii) give compensation of Rs 10 lakh to families of all persons who have died in manholes and septic tanks since 1993.

To diffuse the idea pioneered by SKA, it launched a country-wide march (*yatra*) – the *Bhim Yatra*, which was launched on 10 December 2015 for

125 days covering 30 states and 500 districts. It came to an end on 13 April 2016 on the eve of the 125th birth anniversary of Dr BR Ambedkar and is remembered as a journey of intolerance of the violence, discrimination and violation of constitutional and fundamental rights.

The story of the evolution of the SKA into a people's movement is itself the story of an innovation at work. The organisational values of human dignity, self-respect and equality pervade the work of SKA and percolate into the social innovations it has led. Through a significant social innovation that involved organising *safai karmacharis* across states and districts, articulating a bold vision that upheld their dignity and acknowledging not just the hazardous nature of their work but also the caste implications, SKA has created a transformative movement in the country. The SKA continues to expand both in its geographical reach and in its initiatives of rehabilitating liberated manual scavengers, educating their children and building the Sewerage Workers' Platform and women self-help groups (SHGs) across India. SKA has proven its exclusive commitment to the issues of sanitation workers by bringing out the human perspective of sanitation to the forefront.

As a movement to bring about social change, SKA's focus has centred on organising and mobilising the community around the issues of dignity and rights, accompanied by strategic advocacy and legal interventions. Further, SKA has invested in building awareness of the equality and dignity of every human being, directly confronting issues related to caste and patriarchy. It exemplifies a social innovation in the urban sanitation sector that seeks to bring about a mindset change in the way in which sanitation workers are viewed by the society and the government.

**Jan Sahas:** Jan Sahas started work in 2000. Through networking and campaigns, it has advocated issues of socially excluded communities such as the Dalits, local indigenous communities, manual scavengers and other excluded communities. It is committed to promoting the development and protection of the rights of the communities with a special focus on girls and women by eradicating all forms of bondage, including manual scavenging. Its network is spread across rural and urban areas of 48 districts from the five states of Madhya Pradesh, Uttar Pradesh, Rajasthan, Bihar and Maharashtra in India.

Jan Sahas has made laudable efforts in the sanitation field by empowering adolescent girls and women sanitation workers (especially manual scavengers) to end violence and gender justice, by providing skill development for dignified livelihoods and social entrepreneurship, legal aid for access to justice and reform; supporting education and creating a cadre of paralegals to build survivors as leaders, and empowering communities through capacity and organisation building.

In 2001, Jan Sahas launched Rashtriya Garima Abhiyan (RGA) as a national campaign for the eradication of manual scavenging and comprehensive rehabilitation of manual scavengers in India. Ashif Shaikh led the campaign at the national level with networking partners and the Ministry of Social Justice and Empowerment, for the identification of manual scavengers and their rehabilitation. It was due to the efforts of RGA that the state governments of Madhya Pradesh, Maharashtra, Rajasthan, Bihar and Uttar Pradesh recognised the need for the liberation and rehabilitation of scavengers and made several efforts in that stride (Rashtriya Garima Abhiyan, 2011).

On 30 November 2012, RGA started a nationwide march, 'Maila Mukti Yatra', from Bhopal for the total eradication of manual scavenging. As part of the march, RGA launched a mobile campaign demanding a total eradication of the inhuman slavery of manual scavenging by extending support to the Maila Mukti Yatra. Around 10,000 liberated women participated in the *yatra*, appealing to another 50,000 manual scavengers to stop the practice. It spread to 200 districts and 18 states within 63 days (Rashtriya Garima Abhiyan, 2013).

Following that, RGA launched another campaign, 'Knock the Door', on 12 August 2013 from New Delhi for early passage of the legislation and inclusion of demands on rehabilitation and total elimination of manual scavenging in the Indian Railways. Through this campaign, women liberated from manual scavenging knocked on the doors of Parliamentarians and appealed to them to enact the bill (Dalit Network Netherlands, 2013).

**Chintan:** Chintan is an example of an organisation that enables the proactive participation of rag pickers and waste collectors from the informal recycling sector for ensuring equitable and sustainable production, consumption of materials and waste disposal. Chintan's programmes for waste pickers, called the 'Safai Sena', employ those who collect waste from households in the NCR and further incubates an association of 12,000 waste pickers, small traders, itinerant buyers and recyclers from three states (Chintan, 2021). Also, they are involved in providing professional-level waste and e-waste management across residential areas and with over 12 bulk waste generators (ibid.). Furthermore, they have rolled out education programmes to phase out child labour from waste picking, and mainstream children, particularly girls, into schools and help them stay in school.

Chintan has conducted advocacy campaigns, capacity building of those engaged in recycling and awareness generation on the need for reduced consumption and better waste management. Over the years, it has converted waste into social wealth by creating and facilitating green jobs in the waste sector, research and advocacy for better urban policies, organising the informal sector for self-representation and eliminating child labour in the sector.

### Policy and research-oriented work

**Centre for Policy Research (CPR):** Over the last seven years, the water and sanitation team of Scaling City Institutions for India (SCIFI), nested at CPR, has worked on issues and challenges faced by formal and informal sanitation workers to examine how these might be related to technology, service delivery models, questions of institutions, governance, finance and socio-economic dimensions. The SCIFI programme has engaged in research on manual scavengers, documented practices of manual and mechanical cleaning of sewers and septic tank emptiers, explored institutional responses to these practices and organised talks, webinars and podcasts to strengthen knowledge and support national, state and city authorities to develop policies and programmes for interventions with the goal of increasing access to safe and sustainable sanitation in both urban and rural areas.

Through its work, CPR has contributed to an improved understanding of the need to address manual scavenging through sanitation policy briefs on SRMS to strengthen the evidence base. A research project has been undertaken in Punjab (Ludhiana and Fatehgarh Sahib districts) to track the progress and assess the effectiveness of the SRMS scheme. Additionally, CPR has proactively sought opportunities to strengthen the engagement between activists and policymakers and implement agencies on manual scavenging and faecal sludge management (FSM). This effort has been further developed through a sustained engagement with the SKA, a leading network organisation of sanitation workers. As discussed earlier, SKA had filed a PIL to seek directions from the Supreme Court for the complete prohibition and elimination of manual scavenging. SKA sought CPR's support in organising the case documentation, which included perusing several hundred documents filed by various parties in the decade-long period when the case remained in court. The documents from various state governments and local authorities were reports and commitments to undertake future action, which could be followed up by activists and others working in the field. Following these discussions, CPR created an annotated database of these documents for SKA.

It was during the COVID-19 pandemic that CPR launched a rapid research study, 'Invisible Sanitation Workers @ Covid 19 Lockdown: Voices from 10 Cities', to delve deeper into issues sanitation workers faced during the lockdown (CPR, 2019). The study explored their work condition, which was jeopardised across the country with the outbreak of COVID-19 and the extent to which these frontline workers were exposed to a wide range of both social and occupational vulnerabilities. The study underscored pre-existing vulnerabilities of frontline workers that were exacerbated during the pandemic lockdown and the need to strengthen preparedness and response measures to safeguard these invisible frontline sanitation workers.

**Participatory Research in Asia (PRIA)**: PRIA uses participatory and narrative-centric approaches to address the issues of sanitation workers and their surrounding relations of power. It is through this approach that people come together to change prevailing power dynamics. Such a change is critically required, considering the lack of power omnipresent in the lives of sanitation workers in their workplaces as well as across society. It focuses on narratives that come from the lives of sanitation workers, especially women, which are critical to fostering empathy among the state and society and respecting them as indispensable cogwheels of India's sanitation system.

The seminal participatory research study, 'Bodies of Accumulation – A Study on Women Sanitation Workers', under the 'Engaged Citizens, Responsive City' (ECRC) (PRIA, 2018a) project supported by the European Union, brought out the intersectionality of caste, gender and informality that cumulatively and additively aggravate the injustice, insecurity and indignity of women sanitation workers. The study reverberated that women sanitation workers were subjected not only to wage disparity or occupational hazards but also to the established patriarchal attitudes and behaviour in their homes, communities and workplaces.

PRIA's work in this arena offers a powerful example of how social knowledge – in this case the awareness of caste, class and gender fault lines – can impact the way sanitation workers are received, understood and accepted in that light. Other relevant works by PRIA on sanitation workers are 'Research Report: Dusting the Dawn – A Study on Women Sanitation Workers in the Muzaffarpur, Bihar' (PRIA, 2018b) and 'Lived Realities of Women Sanitation Workers in India – Insights from a Participatory Research Conducted in Three Cities of India' (PRIA, 2019).

**Urban Management Centre (UMC):** Through technical support to the GOI and the State Government of Odisha, UMC contributed to guiding government and non-government functionaries through manuals, tool books and videos on ensuring the safety and dignity of sanitation workers. UMC has been extending relentless support to the government in developing handbooks, reckoners, manuals and video modules on sanitation workers for functionaries at the city, state and national levels to improve its service delivery. UMC has published a handbook to guide sanitation workers on the correct use of personal protective equipment (PPE), which broadly talks about the correct process of wearing and removing PPEs, their maintenance as well as disposal (UMC, 2020). UMC has developed another knowledge product guiding ULBs to ensure the safety and dignity of sanitation workers titled 'Ensuring Safety of Sanitation Workers – A Ready Reckoner for Urban Local Bodies' (MoHUA, 2021).

UMC is supporting the State Government of Odisha by setting up dedicated technical support units at the state and city levels for effective implementation of the Garima Scheme. The scheme strives to enforce Articles 14, 17, 21 and 47 of the Constitution of India (Ministry of Law and Justice Legislative Department, 2020) by regulating the sanitation sector, improving the working environment, providing identity to sanitation workers, and enabling social and financial benefits to sanitation workers and their families.

**Water Aid India (WAI) and Centre for Equity Studies (CES):** WAI, CES and other organisations have been undertaking studies on the most inhuman and undignified forms of sanitation work prevalent in India. The studies have revealed how social stigma and isolation as well as unimaginable health hazards are accrued to manual scavenging. A large number of sanitation workers die, especially those who repair and clean sewer lines, in the absence of any critical safety measures and/or technologies.

In 2018, under the 'Strengthening Rule of Law and Advancing Rights and Freedoms of Manual Scavengers in India' – European Commission – European Instrument of Democracy and Human Rights (EC-EIDHR) funded project, WAI, CES and the Association for Rural and Urban Needy (ARUN) conducted studies to understand different dimensions of manual scavenging. The studies stressed upon the degree of occupational health risks involved, including leptospirosis, skin problems and respiratory system problems, as well as alienation from health services. Further, studies revealed how women engaged in manual scavenging often faced added challenges such as discrimination by employers, government officials and administrators, the public as well as their own community and families; the denial of rights; violence, abuse and sexual harassment (WaterAid India, 2019).

**SWaCH, a Waste Collectors' Cooperative:** In 1993, waste pickers and itinerant waste buyers in Pune and Pimpri Chinchwad came together to form Kagad Kach Patra Kashtakari Panchayat (KKPKP), a membership-based trade union that aimed to establish and assert waste pickers' contribution to the environment, their status as workers and their crucial role in the solid waste management (SWM) of the city. KKPKP has more than 9,000 members, 80 percent of whom are women from socially backward and marginalised castes.

In 2005, KKPKP launched a pilot programme in collaboration with the Pune Municipal Corporation (PMC), SWaCH PMC, where waste pickers were integrated with door-to-door waste collection (DTDC). This paved the way for SWaCH, a wholly owned workers' cooperative as a pro-poor, public–private partnership to undertake such work. The SWaCH DTDC model was based on the recovery of user fees from service users and the provision of infrastructure and management support from the municipality, which was also to play an enabling role. The pilot was implemented in collaboration with the Department of Adult Education, SNDT Women's University, in 2006, and enabled 1,500 waste pickers to become service providers for DTDC of waste from 1,25,000 households in Pune city.

In 2008, the doorstep collection work was institutionalised under the aegis of SWaCH, which was specifically registered for this purpose. With time, SWaCH diversified into verticals as well as extended its service delivery to another city. Besides SWaCH PMC, there is also the SWaCH Plus programme, which focuses on livelihood upgradation and income enhancement activities of waste management such as V-Collect events where citizens can dispose of their unused household items; composting; e-waste collection and disposal through the correct channels; making and selling stabilisation tank (ST) disposal bags (for disposal of sanitary pads, cloth or napkins); awareness raising events; etc. Following this, in 2018, the waste pickers of SWaCH expanded their footprint to reach a total of 1,50,000 slum properties, reducing the number of containers and chronic spots in the city significantly. The cooperative covers over 70 percent of the city, ensuring daily segregated waste collection from citizens' doorsteps while generating sustainable livelihoods for one of the poorest and most marginalised social sections.

The KKPKP union has helped waste pickers demand their rights and dues, and pushed for better working conditions by integrating waste pickers into the waste collection/disposal system. This initiative considerably improved their conditions of work and upgraded their livelihoods, effectively bridging the gap between households and the municipal waste collection service, thereby serving the waste pickers' interest in upgrading their livelihood as well as the municipality's interest in sustainable SWM.

## 5. CONCLUSION

Sanitation work, especially waste management, remains the most hazardous, underpaid and undignified work, with workers suffering discrimination, ostracism, oppression and exploitation. The edifice of the caste system in India has perpetuated the drudgery and dehumanising work of sanitary workers for ages. Despite legal provisions banning manual scavenging in the country, the practice has not waned, reflecting the apathy of the government and policymakers, as well as of India's citizens, leading to the growing invisibility of sanitary workers. Hazardous work conditions, continued oppression, hidden identities and the informal nature of the work exacerbate their vulnerabilities and eschew their access to social security benefits, including safety and dignity.

Various civil society organisation (CSOs), through innovative approaches to raising consciousness among sanitary workers, citizens, the law and policymakers, have drawn attention to the plight of sanitary workers, taking action to make their lives a little more dignified. Continuous assailing of dominant practices of oppression towards sanitary workers and shaking the consciousness of policymakers to bring change into the lives of sanitary workers have been central to social innovations practised by CSOs even with the launch of SBM. Though the mission aimed to eradicate manual scavenging, many state governments and ULBs did not have a database of manual scavengers to link them with various schemes owing to the informal nature of the work and lack of political will to acknowledge their presence. CSO engagement with the government through policy, research and activism has enabled policymakers to deepen their engagement on the issues of safety and dignity of sanitary workers.

Movements of *safai karamchari* to meet unmet needs of dignity, protection, recognition and safety nets while engaging in a hazardous occupation could find a place in policy circles owing to social innovations ushered in by CSOs, deeply embedded in principles of organisation building and participation.

Empowering, protecting the rights and ensuring the safety and dignity of sanitary workers can be achieved through multistakeholder engagement.

On the one hand, the role of the government to develop and implement policies and regulations to protect the interest and safety of sanitary workers is paramount; while on the other hand, the continuous engagement of CSOs in carrying out social innovations to inform policies remains pivotal.

Carrying forward the idea of the centrality of civil society engagement in innovations around urban sanitation, the next chapter on 'Innovative Technology: Connecting the Disconnect' argues that sanitation technologies cannot be viewed in a social vacuum. It is only when civil society proactively links technology with the felt needs of the community that its impact is multiplied.

# 6 Innovative Technology in Urban Sanitation

## Connecting the Disconnect

## 1. INTRODUCTION

This chapter seeks to examine how technical innovations led by civil society organisations (CSOs) are shaping the recent mainstream response to unmet social problems in the sphere of urban sanitation. It discusses how appropriate technologies developed and piloted by CSOs are addressing sanitation challenges of urban areas in general and the urban poor in particular through cost-effective, context-specific, affordable, environment-friendly and responsive solutions in India. Through case studies wherein CSOs have applied innovative technologies to address sanitation challenges, this chapter underlines the relevance of unpacking and understanding technological solutions as social and environmental good in meeting the unmet needs of the urban poor.

Technological innovation has transformed the way of life across the world since early pre-history. Technologies developed since the industrial revolution shape modern life today and have made a significant contribution to economic prosperity, longevity and quality of life. Modern urban habitats and their constant growth owe much to technical innovation in urban sanitation. Since the first modern sewerage systems were put in place in European cities in the middle of the 19th century, such as London and Hamburg, sanitation technologies have evolved as they spread across the globe. As discussed in Chapter 1, there has been constant and increasing attention paid to sanitation in the Global South; and ever since sanitation technology has also evolved to meet the circumstances of needs in these southern countries. Generations of CSOs have been developing these technologies appropriate to the rapidly changing and lower affordability contexts of these geographies.

The concept of innovation has evolved separately in different technical traditions such as technological studies, medical sciences, mathematics and engineering (Hellstrom, 2004). Rather than following a set sequence, a technological innovation process emerges from complex adaptive systems involving many actors and institutions. Barriers are bound to arise at all stages of innovation, from the invention of technology through its selection,

DOI: 10.4324/9781003197102-6

production, adaptation, adoption and retirement (Anadon et al., 2016). Scholars like Ogburn (1964) identified technology as the fundamental driver of social change, which comes through three-pronged processes, invention, discovery and diffusion and has had far-reaching effects on human relationships (Mutekwe, 2012).

Establishing a mutually reinforcing relationship between technical innovation and social needs is essential for the acceptance and diffusion of any technological innovation. Further, when appropriate technologies are linked to the specific needs of the community, they can be defined as social innovation. In this case, regarding the sanitation needs of the urban poor and other marginalised groups, appropriate technology can address needs, which had gone unmet in the past under the application of traditional technologies. Scholars like Mendoza and Thelen (2008) echoed how the impact of technology is enhanced when it is linked with 'pro-poor' innovations, further referring to products and services that cater to essential needs such as healthcare, housing, food, water and sanitation for impacting human development. Technology when used to solve social and environmental problems can be called social technology, which is defined as technologies that present simple, low-cost and easily applicable solutions that generate social impact in fields as diverse as education, agriculture, health, the environment and leisure (Soares, 2020).

In the subsequent sections, recent exemplars of technological innovations in toilet technologies in the urban sanitation domain are discussed from development organisations such as Centre for Urban and Regional Excellence (CURE), Nidan, Gramalaya and Shelter Associates. Thereafter, another set of cases of innovation in the field of wastewater management by Consortium for Decentralised Wastewater Treatment Systems (DEWATS) Dissemination Society (CDD), Centre for Science and Environment (CSE) and others are critically analysed. Each case study is diagnosed with the question of appropriate technology to support social innovation – i.e., technology that is cost-effective, context-specific, affordable, environment-friendly and responsive to the social needs of the vulnerable sections of the population. Moreover, as per Ogburn's classification, they also demonstrate novelty and diffusion.

## 2. RECENT TECHNOLOGICAL INNOVATIONS PURSUED BY CSOs IN URBAN SANITATION

The sanitation sector has emerged as an exemplary case for pro-poor, social and technological innovations, which have demonstrated vast social and environmental impacts. Uneven diffusion of technologies can become a source of perceived social exclusion (Silvestre & Neto, 2014), and the technological legitimacy of any sanitation service model is anchored strongly by its social attributes (Hall et al., 2014).

Ramani, SadreGhazi and Gupta (2017), in their analysis of innovation in Indian sanitation technologies, point out that to enhance the positive social impact of pro-poor innovations, the focus must be not only on the management of technology but also on the management of social impact. The long-term impact is jointly determined by the true intention of the social enterprise, its capabilities and the nature of contextual challenges. One of the goals of social enterprise is to create, diffuse and sustain innovations, i.e., make new offerings to the community that generate social and/or environmental value and address underserved needs (ibid.).

As discussed in Chapter 1, the sanitation situation in urban India has been improving, albeit slowly, and the focus of CSOs, therefore, has also been shifting to pursue solutions for the continuing unmet needs. Cognizant of the implications, conversations in urban sanitation have expanded beyond toilet infrastructure to safe containment, desludging, treatment and reuse of human waste. There have been continuous efforts in bringing technological developments across various components of the sanitation value chain. As an example, even today there are only a few proven technologies available for environmental sanitation through faecal sludge (FS) treatment, most of which are adopted from wastewater treatment systems (NITI Aayog – NFFSM Alliance, 2021).

CSOs have also focused on technological innovation in urban sanitation, which has directly helped in bringing about a difference in the quality of social lives of people less privileged. The importance of appropriate technology as a cost-effective, locally applicable solution in the context of sanitation across toilet technologies and wastewater treatment models has been very valuable as the sustainable development goal (SDG) target for sanitation has become more ambitious than the millennium development goals (MDGs), as discussed in Chapter 1, and now targets universal coverage of 'safely managed sanitation'.

The technological innovations discussed in the next section focus on providing facilities to train, design and apply research and development along with knowledge management, to meet these social and ecological needs. Table 6.1 maps various socio-environmental technological innovations led by CSOs across the sanitation value chain, including toilet technologies and faecal sludge management (FSM) entailing technical interventions, beginning from the way interfaces are built at the point of generation of excreta to its containment, conveyance, treatment and, finally, safe disposal.

## 3. TECHNOLOGICAL INNOVATION IN URBAN SANITATION: CSO CASES

The cases discussed below illustrate how various CSOs developed technological innovations to meet specific demands of the local context and demonstrated that social and technological innovations need to work hand in hand. The cases examine technological innovations in toilet technologies, decentralised wastewater treatment systems, decentralised wastewater management, low-cost cluster septic tanks (CSTs) and faecal sludge treatment plants (FSTPs), among others, all of which were developed to meet the social

*Table 6.1* Urban sanitation solutions from various CSOs

| CSOs | Technological solutions in urban sanitation |
| --- | --- |
| **Containment** | |
| Gramalaya | Eco-san toilet |
| Centre for Urban and Regional Excellence | Low-cost cluster septic tank |
| Shelter Associate | Child-friendly designs and biodigesters |
| **Collection & transportation** | |
| Bandicoot | Mechanised desludging |
| Blue Water Company | Double-boosting pumping station |
| **Waste treatment** | |
| Centre for Science & Environment | Decentralised wastewater treatment system |
| Consortium for DEWATS Dissemination (CDD) Society | Decentralised wastewater treatment system |
| TIDE Technocrats | Faecal sludge treatment plant (pyrolysis technology) |
| WASH Institute | Mobile faecal sludge treatment unit |
| **Monitoring tool for better planning** | |
| eGov Foundation in partnership with Centre for Policy Research | FSM digit platform |
| Centre for Urban and Regional Excellence | SAMMAN, GIS-based planning tool |
| Shelter Associate | GIS-based mapping, planning and monitoring |
| TIDE Technocrats | Web-enabled monitoring system, SaniTrack |

*Source*: Authors

and ecological needs with low-cost and environment-friendly technologies for urban sanitation.

## Technological solutions in containment

**Gramalaya – Eco-san toilets:** Gramalaya has been working in the sanitation sector for more than three decades and has successfully demonstrated sanitation solutions with various demographic conditions covering rural, urban, coastal and local indigenous areas. In the space of sanitation technologies, it has been advocating a different kind of low-cost toilet model, also known as eco-san toilets, which are affordable and acceptable by communities depending upon the local situation and willingness of the people.

The sanitation technologies that Gramalaya found to be appropriate for use draw on a range of reinvented or recreated toilet technologies and models. It is not so much the invention of new technologies but the selection and showcasing of context-specific and appropriate technologies through its Centre for Toilet Technology and Training at its rural headquarters in Kolakudipatti Village, Thottiam Block, Tiruchi district (Tamil Nadu).

Gramalaya places heavy emphasis on low-cost, location-specific and acceptable technologies. Accordingly, the designs are constructed by community members of their own accord and depending on their socio-economic status, with the support of field staff working on the project. It has combined the construction of twin leach-pit toilets, eco-san toilets, toilets made with septic tanks and community toilets – all duly field tested from the rural context with urban contextualisation on the social side, such as community-managed pay-and-use systems, and toilets for crèches and schools. In showcasing more than 24 toilet models, Gramalaya's training centre has become the first of its kind technology park with designs ranging from leach-pit latrines to eco-sans, community toilets and toilets for schools and mid-day meal centres. The centre displays different successful toilet models requiring different levels of water usage and suitable for various geographical features. Over the last 30 years, Gramalaya's experience in this field has given birth to many successfully field-tested models. A working model of eco-san toilets has been explained in Box 6.1.

---

**Box 6.1 Eco-san toilets from Gramalaya**

Gramalaya has constructed leach-pit toilets and pit latrines using locally available materials. In some operational areas, however, such as in tsunami-affected coastal areas, it has introduced eco-san toilets. These toilets are welcomed by the fisherfolk communities in Nagapattinam district of Tamil Nadu. The successfully field-tested models have been tried out in the water-logged regions of the Cauvery delta in Tiruchirappalli district. Communities like the Varadharajapuram and Thirunarayanapuram villages in Thottiyam block have enthusiastically welcomed them. Though these toilets are expensive when it comes to construction, the long-term benefits of using them outweigh these costs. Nearby communities have also welcomed the eco-san toilets, both in the coastal and in the delta regions.

These toilets are constructed above the ground level with two chambers and two squat holes with urine separation facilities. This way, the wash water is diverted to the kitchen garden and prevented from mingling with human faeces. The urine separated from the toilet is stored or drained using a mud pot. Alternate chambers are used, and once filled, they can also be used as manure in the agricultural fields after one year. Gramalaya constructed 335 eco-san toilets during 2006–2010, which have been used by the communities extensively without any technical problems. These toilets are water-saving and eco-friendly models with more possibilities for extending to other areas with similar needs. In the coming years, Gramalaya hopes that more such eco-san models would be promoted on the basis of research studies and demands from local communities.

*Source*: Gramalaya (n.d. a)

It combines the technical solutions in toilet models developed by its centre with community-managed micro-finance for different sanitation models with a child and women-friendly approach that encourages marginalised communities to invest in creating a context where toilets will not only be constructed in urban slums but also used and managed at the local level, making the community the primary stakeholder in the process. It is the ability to embed it in a social context and form networks and alliances across different sectors that formed the core of the technological efforts introduced by Gramalaya in the area of urban sanitation.

**CURE – Cluster Septic Tank (CST):** CURE has designed the CST which consists of home toilets, a shared septic tank and a DEWATS. Toilets constructed at home are to be linked through a manhole to a simplified sewer system that will carry the waste to the CST. The CST itself acts as a large septic tank with baffle walls to treat the sludge from home toilets and has a retention capacity of a year, after which it needs to be cleaned. The overflow from the CST is treated by the DEWATS, and the treated water is stored in tanks and is available for reuse.

The CST has proven to be a low-cost, de-engineered solution installed in partnership with people in Safeda Basti and Savda Ghevra, Delhi, and Kuchhpura, Agra. It has offered a new template for in-house sanitation services in unplanned urban fringes, bringing sanitation to even the poorest of households.

---

**Box 6.2 Decentralised wastewater treatment system in Kachhpura, Agra, from CURE**

In 2010, to counter the sanitation challenge, CURE constructed a DEWATS in Kachhpura, with the support of the London Metropolitan University and Water Trust, UK. The aim of this project was to improve the quality of lives of people living in informal communities by providing better access to sanitation services and sustainable livelihoods linked to tourism. According to CURE, 'Community-led sanitation initiatives included the construction of household, school and community toilets, a decentralised wastewater treatment system, and solid waste management service improvements'.

The DEWATS was constructed along 100 metres within the Kachhpura stormwater drain to treat 50 kilolitres (kL) of wastewater per day. With zero energy consumption, this system treats black water to bring down its biochemical oxygen demand (BOD) levels from 300 to below 30 by using gravity flow, anaerobic underground tanks and bioremediation with plants. Its five chambers included a filter chamber to filter debris, a septic tank for primary treatment, a baffle filter reactor for secondary treatment, a reed bed system for the tertiary process and an underground sump for storage. The DEWATS treated 50 kL of dirty water daily, before discharging into the river. Residents reused the treated water for non-drinking needs and urban agriculture – nudging a shift from urban sewage-based farming to treated water agriculture.

Since its installation, the DEWATS, a first of its kind in Agra as well as in the state of Uttar Pradesh, has significantly improved the health of residents besides creating a model for de-engineered development that can be replicated. Its impact was visible in its replication when it became the basis for the development of the Taj East Drain Improvement Plan for wastewater treatment.

*Source*: CURE (n.d.)

**Shelter Associates (SA) – Toilet Solutions:** In 1993, SA started its work on urban sanitation on the premise that access to household toilets is the necessary condition for a nation to achieve open defecation free (ODF) status. The innovative approach it adopted came out of addressing the real data gap to deliver appropriate solutions and involved the community in designing and maintaining the block and individual toilets.

SA fosters strategic partnerships with urban local bodies (ULBs) in the cities where it operates. As part of this inclusive approach, therefore, its data knowledge is shared with municipal corporations which could carry out more micro-level interventions without having to rely on inadequate secondary data. SA has worked with municipal corporations of Pune and Sangli Miraj to provide community-led sanitation solutions using an inclusive approach. They have also constantly tried to create small loop treatments by installing biodigesters, especially in public toilets.

---

**Box 6.3 Community toilet in Sangli Wadi from Shelter Associate**

The Community-Led Sanitation Programme (2001) at Sangli (Maharashtra) in western India has assisted around 3,500 households across 12 informal settlements in the city to gain access to adequate sanitation facilities. The initiative was a partnership between the local government (Sangli Miraj Kupwad Municipal Corporation), international agencies (USAID, Indo-US FIRE-D, Cities Alliance), an NGO (SA) and a community-based organisation (Baandhani).

Sangli Wadi is a small settlement of 60 families, mostly employed as agricultural wage labourers. The settlement's location is far away from the city's sewerage network. The degree of community interest reinforced its suitability for a community toilet project. The existing community toilets had no provision for children, resulting in increasing open defecation (OD) in and around the communities. This practice made the outspread of diseases like diarrhoea extremely common.

The community-led design process, facilitated by SA, resulted in a toilet design that included separate facilities for men and women, squatting pans for children, a caretaker's house and a biogas energy system. The user charges paid for the caretaker's salary, and the integrated biogas energy system provided the caretaker with fuel for cooking and lighting. The installation of community toilets was carried out with beneficiary communities who had either employed a caretaker or maintained the toilets themselves. The community toilets in Sangli Miraj included accommodation for a caretaker and a biogas system. The biogas system converted the gases generated by human excreta into a fuel source for the caretaker.

*Source*: Shelter Associate (2008)

From initially being involved in building community toilets, SA has adopted a vision for a 'One Home – One Toilet'. This model is well aligned with the GOI's Swachh Bharat Mission (SBM) initiative launched in 2014 for reducing the incidence of OD and associated violations of a person's health, safety and dignity.

### Technological solutions in emptying and transportation

To promote non-hazardous cleaning and reduce human intervention through more efficient cleaning of manholes, **Bandicoot**, a robotic machine has been developed by Gen Robotics as a socio-technology innovation. This technological solution constitutes a small robot, which cleans manholes and sewers using its arms to lift the lid, clear blockages and check the quantity of poisonous gas inside the manhole. It is also a training assistance for better user experience and easy rehabilitation of sanitation workers.

Similarly, to address the inaccessibility cum manual scavenging issue, Blue Water Company (BWC) developed a technology called a 'Double Boosting Pumping Station'. The technology, first deployed in Leh, is a simple, low-cost method for emptying septic tanks in very narrow streets. It allows a booster pump to be attached to the existing pump mounted on the cesspool emptier vehicle. This helps to increase the reach of the vehicle by two times and requires less investment, only involving the procurement of the pump and the fittings. With its increased reach, this solution is especially useful in hilly terrains and suitable for inaccessible areas with narrow lanes and can further the fight against manual scavenging (NITI Aayog – NFFSM Alliance, 2021).

*Technological solutions in waste treatment*

**CSE – Decentralised Wastewater Treatment (DWWT):** CSE works towards using scientific and research-based facts and promotes DWWT as the wastewater treatment solution for sustainable environment management. The technological efforts of CSE in the field of urban sanitation are rooted in its larger vision of sustainable development that makes it impossible to separate this issue from the central issue of management of water resources. The basic intertwining of sanitation with a much wider 'participatory, efficient and sustainable water management' paradigm is integral to any technical solution in the urban sanitation space. The approach here is to include wastewater treatment or management and FSM within the sanitation issue and link it to the overall issues of environmental pollution. At the core of this approach has been the response to an old problem of neglecting on-site waste management like septic tanks and linking it with the larger sanitation issue.

While the social context of the technology has been kept alive, CSE has used technological solutions that are biological. While the technology is not new, the uniqueness lies in how this technology was used for learning and adapting to the social context. Various methodologies were experimented with, culminating in what has come to be known as the DWWT system.

This system, promoted and implemented by CSE, has used innovative technology and design that has been cognizant of context and geographical variations. Mainstreaming the DWWT system has been a key concern for CSE. CSE's DWWT system uses 'soil biotechnology', a green technology for water purification using a natural, novel high-efficiency oxidation process that combines sedimentation, infiltration and biodegradation. The system also consists of coarse or fine screen chambers/grit chambers for preliminary treatment, treated water tanks, piping, pumps and electrical and civil works. This system also has a bioreactor, which is constructed from reinforced cement concrete (RCC)/stone masonry or soil bunds.

> The bioreactor consists of an underdrain which is covered with layers of different size gravels, coarse and fine sand, culture, media, additives and bio indicators. It consists of microbial culture (native micro flora, geophagus earthworms) required for breaking down and bioconversion of the sewage. Green plants particularly with tap root system act as bio indicators. To avoid leaching of partially treated wastewater into aquifer and to provide a firm foundation for construction soling is done. This is done with stone aggregates of random sizes between 50-150mm. This is followed by fabrication, assembling, fixing and testing of polyvinyl chloride (PVC) network is done on the top of bioreactors and for the under drain.
>
> (CSE, 2014)

The system works by screening and removing grit before water percolates through trenches (containing gravel) and is collected/stored in a collection tank.

After piloting and prototyping the DWWT system as part of the holistic approach to sanitation, the challenge for any social innovative idea is how to scale it up. CSE has implemented the DWWT system in areas of high visibility for 'high impact' with the hope that it will encourage others to implement similar systems and, therefore, scale up the reach of DWWT. It is important to note that CSE's campus in the Qutub Institutional Area in Delhi and its new training campus in Alwar, Rajasthan, are both water-neutral campuses that use the DWWT system. CSE has supported institutions like the Delhi Jal Board (DJB), the National Environmental Engineering Research Institute (NEERI) and the Indian Institute for Technology (IIT) – Jodhpur to put in place DWWT systems.

**CDD Society – DEWATS:** CDD Society is a not-for-profit organisation, which innovates, demonstrates and disseminates decentralised, nature-based solutions for the conservation, collection, treatment and reuse of water resources and management of sanitation facilities.

CDD uses DEWATS, developed with support from Bremen Overseas Research and Development Association (BORDA), for the treatment and management of water by adopting various technologies. DEWATS consists of on-site treatment without chemicals and technical energy inputs and is, therefore, low maintenance.

DEWATS is a nature-based technology and approach to treating wastewater. The approach emphasises the building of many small-scale systems in place of a centralised large system to treat wastewater close to the point of generation, enabling treated water to be effectively reused for gardening and toilet flushing. Simply designed using natural bacteria, plants and gravity instead of electricity and chemicals, this technology has adapted various technologies for conditions where electricity is not reliably available, skilled manpower is hard to come by and mechanical parts that break may never be repaired. This treatment system cannot be switched off intentionally, and it provides state-of-the-art technology at affordable prices. It is also very easy to integrate aesthetically into built environments and is adaptable to a variety of organic wastewater characteristics. By-products of a DEWATS – biogas, nutrient-rich water and sludge – can be reused for cooking, gardening and composting.

In five years, CDD Society has made a concerted effort to strengthen its network and scale up its approach to reach wider client groups. CDD Society and BORDA, supported by Bill and Melinda Gates Foundation (BMGF), built India's first FSTP in Devnahalli, Karnataka, catering to a population of 30,000 by using low-cost, gravity-based biological treatment.

---

**Box 6.4 CDD case study – FSTP in Devanahalli, Karnataka**

**Technology:** Feeding tank with screen chamber, anaerobic digester (biogas digester with stabilisation tank), integrated settler with anaerobic baffled reactor and anaerobic filter (ABR + AF), planted gravel filter (PGF), sludge drying bed (SDB), collection tank (CT)

**Capacity:** 6 m³; **Reuse:** compost, biogas, treated water; **Year of operation:** November 2015

Devanahalli Town Municipal Council (TMC) is the headquarter of Devanahalli Taluk. It is about 39 km northeast of Bangalore city. With the increasing growth of the population in Bangalore city, and given the town's proximity to the Bangalore international airport, the population flux into Devanahalli has also been increasing. This fast growth and lack of proper sanitation facilities in the town are leading to environmental pollution with risks to human health.

CDD Society identified the above problem and proposed to implement a faecal sludge treatment plant (DEWATS) within Devanahalli's municipal limits to treat the sludge from septic tanks and pits of households, commercial establishments and government buildings. The faecal sludge is conveyed to the proposed treatment location through a cesspool vehicle. The proposed DEWATS modules for the FSTP include feeding tank (FT), biogas settler (BGS), stabilisation tank (ST), SDB, integrated settler and ABR with filter chambers, PGF and CT. The plant is maintained by the Devanahalli Town Municipal Council with external support from certain not-for-profit organisations.

*Source*: CDD (2018)

---

CDD has supported the diffusion of technology in many small cities and towns since 2016. Many low-cost, decentralised FSTP systems have been set up across the country, including those at Angul and Dhenkanal in Odisha, as part of 'Project Nirmal' supported by the Centre for Policy Research and Practical Action (PA). This involved covering a population of 70,000–1,00,000 from both cities with this environment-friendly, cost-effective, gravity-based anaerobic digestion technology.

Under Project Nirmal, SCI-FI CPR and Practical Action constructed FSTPs with technical support from CDD. The technology used is anaerobic stabilisation reactor (ASR), unplanted sludge drying bed (UPDB) with DEWATS screen and grit chamber, anaerobic stabilisation reactor, unplanted sludge drying bed, integrated anaerobic baffled reactor and anaerobic filter (ABR + AF), planted gravel filter, collection tank, sand and carbon filter, and pasteurisation unit.

Centre for Policy Research (CPR) and Practical Action, with technical support from CDD Society, demonstrated appropriate, low-cost, decentralised

FSTP and a citywide FSM system at Angul and Dhenkanal in Odisha. Built with passive, low-energy and low-skill technologies, the FSTPs have been in operation for more than two years now and have been consistently meeting environmental regulations and serving urban households.

Project Nirmal was designed and intended to demonstrate the feasibility of a citywide, low-cost decentralisation sanitation system using a nature-based treatment system for small and mid-sized cities and towns in Odisha. With a capacity of 27 kilolitres per day (KLD) in Dhenkanal and 18 KLD in Angul, the FSTPs were built under Project Nirmal using an integrated service contract model with a call centre, desludging private operator and FSTP maintenance. Through the project, the state government and the ULBs demonstrated commitment to urban sanitation service delivery by providing faecal sludge and septage management (FSSM) as one of the solutions for addressing and regulating the indiscriminate disposal of FS. Further, the FS was treated at FSTPs and the by-products were reused, thereby closing the sanitation loop.

Now Dhenkanal FSTP serves rural households. In pursuance of the understanding with the Panchayati Raj Department, Housing and Urban Development Department (H&UDD), UNICEF and CPR, a pilot project for Solid and Liquid Waste Management (SLWM) in rural Dhenkanal is being undertaken. The urban FSSM facilities in Dhenkanal district are being extended to 17 *gram panchayats* within a radius of 10 km of the city in 2021 followed by covering 110 gram panchayats by 2022. To formalise delivery of urban FSSM services, Dhenkanal Municipality and the *gram panchayats* have entered into an Ministry of Urban Development (MoUD) through the Sadar Block, defining a clear set of responsibilities for local bodies and the tariff structure for desludging in rural areas.

CDD Society had established a Centre for Advanced Sanitation Solutions (CASS) in 2011, along with its partners, Rajiv Gandhi Rural Housing Corporation Ltd. (RGRHCL) and the Bremen Overseas Research and Development Association to upgrade and disseminate knowledge on sustainable sanitation solutions. CASS is equipped with facilities to provide training, design, applied research and development besides knowledge management units alongside an interactive exhibition. As the access to a safe and sanitisation environment is considered a basic human need and right, CDD's water treatment systems and decentralised solid waste management interventions were customised for low-income communities and termed Decentralised Basic Needs Service (DBNS). The technical aspects of sanitation space were embedded in a specific social context with handholding techniques and transfer of knowledge to enable low-income communities to both understand and access these technologies.

The consortium has, thus, sought to provide an eco-friendly, low-maintenance and energy-neutral technology suitable for managing a wide range of wastewater at reasonable costs. Over the past decade, CDD Society has grown to become the only sanitation-specific technological institute in India that has implemented the maximum number of DEWATS in Asia. It has been hired by the state governments of Andhra Pradesh and Tamil Nadu as well as the Municipal Corporation of Shimla to solve sanitation and wastewater challenges at the city level.

To make sanitation technologies more affordable, CDD has made decentralisation its key mantra. Additionally, it has widened its scope to septage and FSM. To develop an effective design for septage treatment, a pilot treatment system has been implemented in CASS, which is based within the CDD Society. This treatment system is currently being monitored to develop various design criteria to enable the upscaling of septage treatment methodologies.

Quite evidently, the basic need that triggered CDD's technological solution was the challenge of making treatment systems affordable and bringing down the cost of treatment, which is estimated to range from Rs 14,000 to 25,000 per citizen per city; in addition to operations and other costs, if this were to be a centralised treatment system. There is also the difficulty of scaling up under this centralisation system, as cities grow to connect every household to these pipelines through difficult topography and land-holding issues. DEWATS is based on the notion of building many small systems requiring less pipelines and low operating costs and can be adapted across different urban landscapes.

Like CDD and CSE, there are organisations like **Tide Technocrats** and **Water, Sanitation and Hygiene Institute (WASH Institute)**, who are working extensively in the space of FSM.

**Tide Technocrats Pvt. Ltd.** works in the area of FSM and provides environmentally sustainable technological solutions. Over the years, it has been overseeing the Wai FSTP facility, by monitoring the quality of output and by-products regularly as per standards and sharing the performance report of inlet and outlet information with Wai Municipal Council (WMC). The Wai FSTP was set up by Tide Technocrats Pvt. Ltd., based on the thermal treatment process. It has a 70 KLD capacity and consists of a septage receiving station, holding tank, dewatering unit, pasteurisation unit, dryer and pyrolysis unit and a wastewater treatment unit. The treated liquid from the treatment plant is used for landscaping within the premises and for washing vacuum tankers and solid waste collection vehicles. It is modular, and the size and capacity of the plant can be easily augmented with the existing modular units in future. The overall site is compact, unlike a typical treatment plant with physically oversized units. The plant does not produce any odour and is suitable for varying climatic conditions. With the Wai FSTP, the municipal council has been able to promote a scientific treatment of collected faecal sludge and septage. There has also been an emphasis on the potential of reusing treated water and utilising biochar for landscaping and plantation for future agricultural needs. There has been a significant reduction in the usage of potable water for non-potable purposes as well as in the pollution level of the land, water bodies and rivers. There has also been a significant public health improvement by preventing water-borne diseases such as diarrhoea, dysentery, cholera, jaundice and typhoid, leading to savings on public health expenditure. Additionally, the FSTP has created employment opportunities for semi-skilled local residents. Wai has shown the way to other municipalities on how to operate a compact treatment facility with easy maintenance.

Similarly, the **WASH Institute** is involved in action research to develop innovative sanitation products and comprehensive WASH programmes for communities and schools across rural and urban areas, particularly Mobile Treatment Units (MTUs). An MTU is an on-site faecal sludge treatment (FST) system mounted on the bed of a small truck that treats the effluent of septic tanks. This on-site mobile septage treatment unit works on the concept of solid–liquid separation, sludge thickening and effluent treatment processes. While the liquid is separated from the solid, the effluent passes through the treatment process and disposes of the treated effluent. The operational capacity of the MTU varies from 3,000 to 6,000 litres/hour. The higher flow rate of an MTU, therefore, helps in emptying and treating a greater number of septic tanks per day, bringing down the operational cost of the truck as well as the desludging service fee for customers. The total cost of each MTU is much lower than the septage emptying trucks used by private operators. This on-site technology is easy to operate with its low operational and maintenance costs. Therefore, MTUs attempt to address several barriers to achieving safely managed septic waste; they are financially scalable and are designed to be replicable across geographies.

### Monitoring tools for better planning

**FSM digital platform**: SCI-FI CPR supported e-Government Foundation in developing a National Digital Platform for FSM to assist states and ULBs in managing, monitoring and streamlining FSM service delivery. The two organisations co-developed a concept and scaffolding for the platform. The FSM digital platform aims to assist the state and local governments in exercising effective cost control measures that are especially crucial for FSM, given that operations and maintenance (O&M) costs make up 60–75 percent of total FSM systems' costs. The platform supports data-driven policy decisions on costs, tariffs and additional upgrading requirements and monitoring levels of service for citizen satisfaction. The FSM platform connects citizens with ULBs for better service.

SCI-FI CPR and eGov partnered with the Housing and Urban Development Department (HUDD), State Government of Odisha, to pilot the platform across the state, starting with the urban municipalities of Balasore, Berhampur and Dhenkanal. In Odisha, the FSM digital platform aims to build a digital marketplace to connect citizens with desludging operators through the ULB, allowing citizens to request pit cleaning, service blocked drainage, select operators and give post-collection feedback; while the ULBs enrol, regulate and monitor desludging operators and collect data on pits and septic tanks integrated with property data, along with GIS mapping. The platform has completed its first phase of development and testing in Balasore, Berhampur and Dhenkanal municipalities, enabling citizens in availing and tracking desludging services online, as well as allowing ULBs to track the status of faecal sludge from desludging to disposal at the designated FSTP (as of July 2021).

---

**Box 6.5 SANMAN, a GIS-based planning tool from CURE**

Sanitation Manager or SANMAN is a planning tool developed by CURE that uses a GIS digital platform to layer sanitation data upon city maps for sanitation investment projections for under-serviced populations living in informal and squatter settlements in Indian cities. SANMAN was conceived by CURE to collate data generated from informal settlement communities using community mapping and participatory processes to understand the spatial distribution of services in these areas, as well as the area's proximity to city infrastructure to incubate and innovate simplified sanitation solutions that are equalising, integrating and inclusive.

CURE has successfully collaborated with the municipal corporations and ULBs in East Delhi, North Delhi, Agra, Noida, Dharamshala, Shamli, Shahjhanpur, Jaipur, Ghaziabad, Rourkela, Ajmer, Gopalpur, Muzaffarpur and Bhubaneswar to crowdsource large amounts of spatial and non-spatial data to converge and digitise them to build SANMANs. SANMANs have been combined with various technologies like GIS, Google mobile services, and web-based applications for documentation, analysis and data visualisation. The information system thus developed has supported the smart decisions of these cities to locate new municipal services and allocate, target, optimise resources and manage them effectively.

SANMANs have proven to be very effective in the collection and integration of community data with city data; collation of data dispersed across municipal services to create a citywide information system that is easy to access and use for planning service delivery, which results in improved service delivery and operations; and city savings from reduced redundancy and duplication of efforts and better management of city assets and property. It has also enabled seamless inter-departmental and inter-agency coordination producing convergence, public safety benefits and economies of scale including that from shared data and continued improvement of workflows and optimised use of staff and scarce resources by integrating data with city management systems.

*Source*: CURE (n.d.)

CURE has also pioneered a GIS mapping of solid waste and sanitation resources in several locations near bins, waste hotspots, urinals, public toilets, drains, etc. This has enabled an analysis of these areas with respect to the type of waste generated, volume, community profile, etc., to come up with effective investment and management solutions. CURE's initiative, SANMAN (see Box 6.6 for details), has enabled ULBs to plan investments in areas not adequately serviced, to use their resources efficiently by planning collection routes, connecting toilets to sewerage systems, linking drains to outfalls and monitoring service delivery.

**SA's spatial planning:** SA's experience demonstrates how spatial mapping, social surveys and GIS can be used to ascertain community sanitation priorities and develop feasible technical designs. SA has facilitated access to sanitation in informal settlements by setting up a very robust spatial data platform to mark families who lack access to basic sanitation. It facilitates the construction of community toilet blocks as well as individual toilets. In a unique initiative, it used data collected in partnership with the community by juxtaposing it with Google Maps to create evidence-based plans for sanitation needs, particularly in the areas inhabited by the urban poor. These GIS maps help ensure that the requisite infrastructure (sewage pipes or septic tanks) and toilets are provided in the right location, keeping in mind topography, road access conditions, family characteristics and neighbourhoods. The mapping is further supplemented with survey data collected at the household level and analysed to identify the most vulnerable population and plan targeted interventions. The model emphasises individual toilets as a solution to urban poor sanitation problems and also demonstrates effective community toilet management structures (Shelter Associate, 2008).

**TIDE Technocrats' Sani Track:** Tide Technocrats, Bangalore, has been operating FSTPs and has been primarily responsible for monitoring the quality of output and by-products as per standards and sharing the performance report of inlet and outlet information with WMC for their monitoring purposes. For monitoring desludging service delivery, an online, web-enabled monitoring system called SaniTrack has been developed. Developed by the Centre for Water and Sanitation (CWAS) and Centre for Environmental Planning and Technology (CEPT), SaniTrack consists of a mobile app and web modules, wherein the de-sludger schedules and records daily operations with signatures like in an e-commerce app, allowing city managers to see real-time information on (i) geographical coverage, (ii) schedule progress, (iii) household readiness, (iv) safe conveyance from household to FSTP, (v) customer satisfaction and (vi) use of personal protective equipment (PPE), on a dashboard. The dashboard offers key performance indicators, timeline filters and map-based insights and also allows downloadable data for more detailed analysis. On the other end, SaniTrack simplifies the process of maintaining paper forms by reducing them to clicks, signatures on a screen and automatic location/time crosschecks. These can later also be downloaded in the form of individual reports containing addresses, photographs and signatures, similar to a paper-based form.

Similarly, ULBs in Odisha have installed GPS-based vehicle tracking and monitoring systems in all cesspool vehicles (government-procured and private vehicles) for efficient and accountable desludging operations in the sanitation value chain. This ensures real-time monitoring of operations on the ground and aids greater accountability among stakeholders, especially when coupled with incentive and penalty structures. Real-time monitoring has also improved plant utilisation from an erstwhile 10–20 percent capacity to over 100 percent in some areas (NITI Aayog – NFFSM Alliance, 2021).

## 4. CONCLUSION

This chapter has documented recent technological innovations from containment through low-cost toilets; collection and transportation innovations, wastewater treatment and monitoring, as well as planning tools. The discussion shows that a lack of attention to user considerations can lead to a mere transfer of technology without consideration of appropriateness as well as information to the user putting at risk the long-term usability and sustainability of the technology. It is only where technological advancement meets its social responsibility that the true scope of social innovation is unravelled.

At the heart of India's sanitation problem, therefore, lies the question of 'appropriate' technology – one that is cost-effective, context-specific, affordable, environment-friendly and responsive to the social needs of the vulnerable. A new thinking that links urban sanitation to not just eco-friendly technology but also user-centric tech is being developed along participatory models. It will carry with it the possibility of scaling up without which the urban sanitation problem cannot be resolved. A holistic approach also demands that technical innovations draw on the contributions of local knowledge systems, local wisdom and a wide variety of cultural values.

Several experiences from urban sanitation indicate such a *hybrid* approach. For example, the social innovations of CSE bring together diverse elements such as strengthening the capacities of city officials on preparing city sanitation plans and septage management projects, decentralised wastewater treatment programme within its overall paradigm of promoting sustainable and equitable development. CURE, on the other hand, offers a *hybrid* approach since it combines new technological ideas from its in-house team with community-based solutions and resources to co-design and co-implement interventions.

Case studies have demonstrated that social and technological innovations are predominantly developed and diffused through CSOs and are primarily motivated by the goal of meeting a social need and creating an impact on the ground, cutting across organisational, sectoral and disciplinary boundaries. This intersectionality is a key feature of social innovations as they require finances, authority and ideas to come together. The Shelter Associate and Centre for Policy Research with eGov has brought an inter-sectoral approach so that smart, IT-based solutions can be used for city sanitation planning. CDD has worked with a network of more than 20 like-minded partners across the country to propagate and diffuse the idea of decentralised wastewater management in urban sanitation domain. Due to the intersectionality of different disciplines and sectors in almost all social innovations studied in this research, a set of new relationships between pre-viously disjointed individuals and groups have resulted in the diffusion of ideas, where each innovation has the potential to trigger innovations.

Thus, CSOs have successfully advanced technological innovation by incorporating the pivotal role of social actors who are not only technical experts but also end-users, policymakers, social enterprises, entrepreneurs, political, social, economic and planning institutions. They need to help in translating the benefits of new technologies in sanitation into tangible bene-fits, such as increased safety, affordability, accessibility and even mere avail-ability. It is, thus, an entire process of value generation and value transfer of technological innovations that are converted into social innovation that can effectively eradicate deprivations and bolster capabilities in the sanitation infrastructure.

Building on this chapter that demonstrates how CSOs have used the social innovations approach and draw on appropriate and specific technologies for particular circumstances; the next chapter discusses how CSOs provide platforms for multistakeholder capacity building to help further inclusive sanitation. The same comes out of the realisation that all stakeholders need to embrace change if society is to achieve safe, equitable and sustainable sanitation for all.

# 7 Multistakeholder Capacity Building for Inclusive Urban Sanitation

## 1. INTRODUCTION

Capacity can be defined as the totality of inputs needed by an actor to realise its purposes (Tandon, 2002). This chapter delineates three levels of capacity building: (i) individual level: the leadership and human resources; (ii) institutional level: organisational strategy, structure, technology, processes and culture and (iii) sectoral level: enabling laws, policies and the external environment. For social innovations in the urban sanitation sector to be successful, a well-strategised capacity-building effort of relevant stakeholders is required to address all areas and all levels of capacities. This chapter examines innovative practices of multiple stakeholders on capacity building in urban sanitation with a special focus on capacity building of urban local bodies (ULBs) since these are the designated institutions responsible for delivering the programmes related to urban sanitation as per the XII Schedule of the 74th Constitutional Amendment Act.

The capacity building of ULBs aims to ensure that such institutions can function effectively as institutions of local self-governance. Tandon (2002) provides a useful archetype of capacities that could be relevant to the capacity building of ULBs. The capacity of ULBs can be seen in three distinct, albeit interrelated aspects. First is **intellectual capacity**, which implies the capacity to think, reflect and analyse reality independently and in pursuit of self-defined purposes of local self-governance. The second is **institutional capacity**, which implies procedures, systems, structure, staffing, decision-making, transparency and accountability, planning, implementing and monitoring. It also includes mechanisms for building linkages with other institutions and actors. The third is **material capacity**, which includes material resources, physical assets, funds, systems and procedures to mobilise revenues; access and control physical and natural resources as well as the infrastructure systems and procedures required for adequate management of funds and such infrastructure.

Viewed from this perspective, the capacity of a local body is an examination of its purposes at a given period of its life cycle. Capacity building needs to change over time – it requires an element of diversity and temporal

DOI: 10.4324/9781003197102-7

dynamism. Invariably, the training of individuals is seen as the sine qua non of capacity building through some predetermined package of inputs. However, capacity building comprises a variety of other approaches and processes such as organisational strengthening, institutional learning, exposure, horizontal sharing and solidarity as illustrations of practical, hands-on and experiential learning processes to capacity building. Viewed in this sense, capacity building is a long-term process of strengthening ULBs based on systematic learning of new knowledge, skills and attitudes. Like all learning, the actor herself must see the value of and take responsibility for that learning (Tandon & Bandhyopadhyay, 2003; Tandon & Bandyopadhyay, 2004).

In the Indian context, the overall policies, strategies and resource allocations related to urban sanitation are mainly determined by the union and state governments, while the ULBs are primarily responsible for delivering the programmes. The 74th Constitutional Amendment Act (Part IX-A) of the Indian Constitution envisages ULBs as institutions of local self-governance. The union and state governments are required to devolve appropriate functions, functionaries and finances to the ULBs, but in practice this devolution is uneven. The ULBs have, consequently, remained dependent on the union and state governments for resources and other forms of capacities.

The Swachh Bharat Mission (SBM) and Atal Mission for Rejuvenation and Urban Transformation (AMRUT) – two coveted programmes of the union government on urban water and sanitation – provide critical resources to the ULBs for programme implementation. However, the capacities required for ULBs to design, plan, implement, monitor and assess the programmes sustainably and inclusively are far from adequate.

The urban sanitation programme that works for all in the city across socio-economic classes and all genders would require engagement by multiple stakeholders. Since there has been little precedence for multistakeholder engagement in a city context, the capacities of all stakeholders need to be enhanced to make sanitation services more inclusive. It is, therefore, imperative that capacity-building interventions are planned and implemented for state and local governance institutions, social sector and citizens' organisations as well as private institutions.

This chapter showcases the innovative practices of civil society organisations (CSOs) like Centre for Urban and Regional Excellence (CURE), which has emphasised building capacities of low-income communities and ULBs to engage in participatory planning for Water, Sanitation and Hygiene (WASH) services in several cities. The Centre for Science and Environment (CSE) too has provided capacity-building support to ULB officials and engineers on septage management, municipal solid waste management, planning, designing and decentralising wastewater treatment, water-sensitive urban design and planning, etc., using both classroom and field-based learning methods. Centre for Policy Research (CPR), under its Scaling City Institutions for India (SCI-FI) initiative, has piloted sustainable sanitation service delivery under Project Nirmal at Angul and Dhenkanal in Odisha. It has demonstrated a city-wide sanitation system for small cities by incorporating faecal sludge management (FSM) for on-site sanitation systems and provided simultaneous capacity-building support to these municipalities. This chapter also discusses the innovative practices of Urban Management Centre (UMC), Gramalaya, National Institute of Urban Affairs (NIUA) and Participatory Research in Asia (PRIA) in building capacities of multiple stakeholders in urban sanitation.

## 2. CAPACITY CHALLENGES IN THE URBAN SANITATION SECTOR

Over the decade, concerns around the deficiency in infrastructure and innovation in technologies on issues of sanitation have gained pertinence, while the capacity building of ULBs and state governments has remained an area of neglect in most Indian states and ULBs. It is with the implementation of the 74th Constitutional Amendment Act that ULBs were intended to be empowered and capacitated as decentralised governance institutions for effective devolution of funds, functionaries and functioning of programmes and schemes to the last mile. However, in the given sanitation space, the question remains whether these bodies are capacitated enough to manage the function and whether funds and functionaries are present with the ULBs to play the role effectively.

The progress on sanitation was dismally low at the beginning of the decade.[1] With the introduction of SBM, approximately 6,260,606 household toilets and 615,864 community toilets/public toilets (CTs/PTs) have been constructed in urban areas till the end of the first phase of SBM. The later part of the decade saw a significant number of toilets without a commensurate spread of the sewer network with most of the newly constructed toilets connected to on-site sanitation (OSS) systems[2] across urban areas. In the absence of a well-developed sewer network across cities and villages, 70 percent of the toilets-owning households in 2011 relied on OSS systems. For optimal functionality, these systems require periodic emptying and off-site treatment of the emptied waste before it can be safely disposed of. The amplifying dependence on OSS systems underscores the need for the safe management of faecal sludge. Continued reliance on groundwater sources and the predominance of sporadically serviced on-site sanitation systems due to the absence of a sewerage network and liquid waste treatment facilities in many cities underscore the emphasis on not only toilets but on managing the sanitation value chain. Thus, knowing technology and developing appropriate systems and protocols of monitoring towards addressing issues of recycling and reuse become critically pertinent.

Additionally, over the years, public health and sanitation have gained increased attention from the National Green Tribunal (NGT) on environment protection, which has further necessitated the need for ULBs to enhance capacities and revisit the supply and demand side aspects of capacity building. With 62 percent of total untreated sewage discharged directly into water bodies and 70 percent of faecal sludge left untreated (CPCB, 2019), there was a need for attention on non-sewered sanitation systems and FSSM in the national and state policies and schemes. In that light, AMRUT allowed for septage management investments encouraging states to submit plans for safe and sustainable FSM solutions. Alongside, the National Policy on Faecal Sludge and Septage Management (NFSSM-2017) and FSSM operative guidelines as well as the state policies by 19 states and Union Territories (2018) were published to help scale up approaches to 'safely managed sanitation', especially for urban areas. From just one FSTP in 2014, there are more than 30 FSTPs in operation today, with about 450 FSTPs under consideration and construction.

Overall, across the country, technology options available with the ULBs are limited, and capacity enhancement is needed across the sanitation sector, including for wastewater disposal. The major shortcomings are weak or inadequate institutional structures and poor policy frameworks; lack of political will due to the low prestige of the sector; inadequate and poorly utilised resources; inappropriate approaches, standards and regulations and neglect of consumer preferences. This lack of capacities is reflected in both the elected and the executive wings of the ULBs across sizes and functions. Hence, the ULBs need to urgently address the issue of ensuring standard designs, as well as the operation and maintenance of toilets across the respective municipal areas (Nair & Dwivedi, 2017). Hence, in terms of FSM, this would mean ensuring that waste is safely contained, collected, transported, treated and, wherever possible, reused. This entails awareness generation among the community to adopt safe and hygienic practices and the municipality to embrace appropriate technologies and practices. This in turn would require revisiting the current human resource structure and management arrangements as well as developing appropriate capacity-building inputs.

What emerges as an element of high relevance is the identification of issues and stakeholders who need capacity enhancement in the ULBs. Among the stakeholders that stand very critical are the ULB employees who are involved in the delivery of municipal services over their entire career period extending over several decades. The cadre that is second in importance is the elected councillors who work with municipal committees as a body on the policy front by reviewing administrative proposals. As elected councillors get renewed every five years, their appropriate orientation in respect of municipal challenges, laws and processes seems to be very prominent. An additional noteworthy dimension is the adequate presence of elected women councillors and equipment of all the councillors with an adequate understanding of gender-related issues to enable gender integration in local government policies in the ULBs. A third and important constituent that needs to be added is the citizens towards whom the municipal services are targeted. Citizen participation enhances the quality of governance. Thus, in the long run, there is a need to review and define staff and human resource requirements, considering the focus on sanitation, the new technologies that need to be introduced and the efficient management systems that will have to be put in place, the proposed agenda to engage with both communities and other service providers.

To address the capacity deficits in the ULBs in general and in the sanitation sector in particular, a host of initiatives have been undertaken by the national government, think tanks, academic institutions as well as civil society organisations. The Sanitation Capacity-Building Platform (SCBP) at the NIUA in a seminal publication (NIUA, 2021) summarises the past and existing capacity-building efforts of Ministry of Housing and Urban Affairs (MoHUA) in the following manner:

> Urban sector-wide capacity development initiatives – a combination of urban reforms (financial and administrative) and sector-wise capacity development, linked with the National Urban Sanitation Policy and the JnNURM since 2005 (e.g., programmes like PEARL – Peer Experience and Reflective Learning and CBUD – Capacity Building for Urban Development).
>
> Programme-specific capacity development initiatives linked with the SBM, AMRUT, Smart Cities and NULM[3] from 2015 (e.g., SMARTNET, linked to SMART Cities Programme; ICBP – Integrated Capacity Development Programme linked to AMRUT and later to all the national programmes and CITTIS programme).
>
> Sanitation-specific capacity development initiatives linked with specific sanitation initiatives like the FSSM and the National FSSM Policy 2017 (e.g., Sanitation Capacity Building Platform (SCBP) – a Capacity Development Normative Framework (of process and training modules) and implementation for non-sewered sanitation systems.
>
> Scaled up urban sector-wide digital capacity-competency initiatives using digital platforms since 2020 (e.g., NULP – National Urban Learning Platform; Mission Karamyogi and iGoT Platform).

With the rising pace of urbanisation and cities growing larger and more complex, capacity enhancement is prone to quick depletion. Before we get into the specifics of such a system, we need to understand the concept and the problems that are currently crippling the present minuscule efforts that go into capacity building. In that light, in the sections below, we glance through the work of organisations furthering efforts towards augmentation of capacity building of the ULBs through periodic training, exposure visits and creation of e-learning platforms. Importantly, talking about regular enhanced learning through a range of tools and methods, such as structured training, periodic planning and review workshops, peer learning and knowledge sharing through a learning portal, newsletters and state-level workshops. This also includes interfacing with resource agencies and best practices, sharing technical know-how and providing resource support to the ULBs. Some of the exemplars from the sanitation space are discussed in the sections below.

## 3. INNOVATIONS IN CAPACITY-BUILDING PRACTICES

*Enhancing capacities in city system for data-driven participatory planning: CURE*

A core principle of the CSO, CURE, is to constantly learn from the partnership with communities. Although CURE has in-house planners, engineers and architects, it works with the community to incorporate local knowledge into plans, which are in turn approved only by community consensus. CURE believes that sustainable change will take place only when the community itself sees value in what they are doing; therefore, the demand for change must come from them. This demand can be facilitated by CURE, but the community must see the need for transformative processes to be effective. CURE has also evolved an ecological approach to improving health outcomes with informal settlements becoming part of the solution to urban resilience. Today, CURE has reached out to approximately 114,000 households in 140 informal settlements in various cities where it works.

CURE does not subscribe to a conventional classroom-based training methodology; it believes in sustained handholding support to the city, state and union governments. It works with the project cities to improve the effectiveness of their planning and water and sanitation service delivery, especially in informal communities by helping cities to (a) engage with people; (b) generate and aggregate data and spatialise it and (c) analyse it to determine gaps, target and deliver services, as per norms/community needs and monitor interventions to ensure sustainability.

A ten-year sustained relationship of CURE with the Agra Municipal Corporation has resulted in CURE's ideas on rainwater harvesting, in-situ slum upgrading, provisioning of household toilets, heritage walks and Decentralised Wastewater Treatment Systems (DEWATS) being incorporated into the Agra Smart City plan. Further, CURE's engagement with the East Delhi Municipal Corporation (EDMC) has resulted in the development of ward sanitation plans, the Adarsh Basti Programme, GIS-based sanitation services, etc., to localise the City Sanitation Plan (CSP) at an area level to enable municipal governments to plan and optimise the use of resources more efficiently. Aligned with the SBM, the ward sanitation plans addressed the entire sanitation bandwidth within the functional space of EDMC's solid waste management, public toilets and drainage at the ward level. The ward plans also recommended comprehensive solutions that address all aspects of sanitation – solid waste, drainage and toilets and the sanitation value chain in each of these related to collection, conveyance, decentralised treatment, resource recovery and disposal.

Under the Urban Sanitation Practices and Capacity Enhancement for Scale – USPaCES, an initiative supported by the United States Agency for International Development (USAID) in eight Indian cities, CURE envisioned (a) building local government capacity for participatory planning and service delivery; (b) generating and using community data for planning, implementing and budgeting for sanitation services; (c) demonstrating innovative, replicable, scalable and inclusive processes and models of water and sanitation service delivery in poor communities that can help cities achieve and sustain its goals under SBM and (d) spreading the scale and integration effects by contributing to the attainment of the Government of India's (GOI) other urban missions like AMRUT, Smart Cities and PMAY.[4] USPaCES is an expansion of an existing programme, 'Pani Aur Swachta Main Sajhedari' (PASS), supported by USAID in Delhi and Agra. PASS had aimed to deliver improved and integrated WASH services to poor communities – taps and toilets at home, to ensure equality, better health and enhanced productivity for sustained poverty reduction. CURE does this through innovating and building scalable service delivery models (decentralised solutions such as simplified sewers, slum networking, cluster septic tanks, customised home toilet, financing models, slope restoration and wastewater treatment to prevent flooding, among others).

Additionally, CURE has ventured into developing an IT application designed to quicken, broaden and manage community participation at scale. The application was designed to transform city–citizen engagement from grievance-based to participatory planning. The application was developed on a simple and smart mobile phone (the phone that most poor owned) using an SMS interface (level of phone using capability among poor women) to engage with people. The application had a three-step process: identifying problem spots and sharing with the city, getting connected to concerned officials responsible for complaint redressal and proposing contextual solutions to address these. Interspersed with direct facilitation processes, the application enables poor communities to raise demands, share ideas and be part of the solution using their phones.

### Knowledge and capacity building: CSE

Taking the central idea of social innovation forward – namely how to integrate waste management with sanitation – requires capacity building for sustainable water management at the outset, and in this respect, CSE has embarked on building capacities of key stakeholders. The Ministry of Urban Development (MoUD)[5] has designated CSE as a 'Centre of Excellence' (CoE) for sustainable water management, under the 'Capacity Building of Urban Local Bodies' (CBULB) programme in 2007. The CoE will conduct residential training programmes, seminars/workshops, exposure visits and research to mainstream best management practices aimed at sustainable urban water management in ULBs under the following new key themes: (i) septage management, (ii) urban lake management, (iii) water-sensitive design and planning, (iv) green infrastructure and (v) water efficiency and conservation.

CSE is involved as a knowledge and capacity-building CSO with SBM and the *Namami Gange* – Clean Ganga Programme. Additionally, CSE has held training programmes at its premises and provided handholding and training support to ten ULBs in the Ganga basin. Based on its work, the MoUD invited CSE to submit a proposal on the training of trainers (ToT) on all aspects related to this holistic approach to sanitation. This included septage management, municipal solid waste management, planning and designing decentralised wastewater treatment, water-sensitive urban design and planning, planning eco-cities, green spaces/infrastructure (town planning) and non-motorised transport, etc. The ToTs were supported by the MoUD from the central share of capacity-building grants, indicating how CSE has been able to partner effectively in linking its vision of sanitation with participatory water management.

**Box 7.1 Education and training centre established by CSE**

The Anil Agarwal Environment Training Institute (AAETI), an education and training initiative of CSE, was established to build a constituency and cadre of knowledgeable, skilled and committed environmentalists – from students, decision-makers, field-level practitioners, civil society groups, journalists, lawyers and concerned citizens.

As part of this mandate, AAETI serves as a research, academic and capacity-building hub that conducts several short- and long-term courses and training programmes. Short-term courses range from technical workshops on how to build rainwater harvesting systems and decentralised wastewater treatment structures to policy issues and hands-on training, information management and advocacy. Other training programmes, such as environment impact assessment (EIA), managing urban growth and urban mobility, seek to actively engage with industry representatives and regulators in the country and across the developing world. Over the past four years, AAETI has conducted more than 100 training programmes, training more than 2,500 participants from India and around the world.

AAETI also conducts month-long certificate programmes on environment/development issues aimed at students and the youth. These orientation programmes give students and young development professionals from India and abroad a first-hand experience of Southern perspectives concerning the environment-development debate. The interdisciplinary coursework allows participants to understand and critically evaluate issues that lie at the interface of environment and development, poverty, democracy, equity, justice and culture.

Course modules include environmental governance in India; the state of natural resource management in the country; poverty and the biomass economy; urban growth challenges; industrial trajectory and pollution control and global environmental negotiations, with a focus on climate change. Certificate courses consist of classroom lectures, seminars and several local field excursions, together with innovative, challenging project, individual and/or group work. They also include a week-long field visit to rural India, where meetings with communities serve to illustrate community-led innovations and eco-restoration efforts.

The core faculty for certificate courses are drawn from CSE's experienced research and programme staff, while guest lecturers include development professionals, eminent environmentalists, noted academicians from leading universities, grassroots activists and prominent policymakers, among others.

### Building capacities in small- and medium-sized ULBs in Odisha – Project Nirmal: Scaling City Institutions for India (SCI-FI) of CPR

CPR, under its Scaling City Institutions for India (SCI-FI) initiative, has piloted appropriate and sustainable sanitation service delivery under the Project Nirmal in Udaipur, Rajasthan, and at two other cities in Odisha – Angul and Dhenkanal. Through Project Nirmal, CPR has demonstrated a city-wide sanitation system for small cities by incorporating FSM for on-site sanitation systems. Project Nirmal presented a strong linkage to the market for collection, transportation, treatment, disposal and reuse. A host of areas like research, capacity building, and knowledge management and advocacy, including policy support to the State Government of Odisha (GoO), were included in the project.

Project Nirmal has demonstrated sustainable sanitation service delivery for small towns leading to increased coverage of households and institutions through institutional and financial arrangements and increased private participation. Project Nirmal has not only deepened its policy and research interventions in Odisha but also demonstrated more meaningful engagement with the public, influencers and decision-makers in strengthening the capacities of ULBs, state officials as well as SBM project management units (PMUs) and technical support units (TSUs) in Odisha.

The overall vision of Project Nirmal is the demonstration of appropriate, low-cost, decentralised, inclusive and sustainable sanitation service delivery solutions for two small towns (Angul and Dhenkanal) in Odisha. The project led to improved sanitation access for all households and integration of FSM in the sanitation value chain, by enabling institutional and financial arrangements as well as increased private sector participation.

The project was implemented by Practical Action (PA) and the CPR with support from the Bill and Melinda Gates Foundation, Arghyam, Housing and Urban Development, GoO, and the municipalities of Angul and Dhenkanal (2015–2020). The project aimed to (a) demonstrate the state government's and the ULB's commitment to sanitation service delivery in small towns; (b) develop the capacity of states and cities for effective sanitation service delivery; (c) increase in the number of people in Angul and Dhenkanal with access to better sanitation services; (d) improve city-wide planning approaches for sanitation and (e) demonstrate models for FSM.

Under the capacity augmentation of the ULBs and concerned stakeholders, the following interventions were undertaken to strengthen the institutional mechanisms to ensure effective coordination and collaboration, while building awareness of roles and responsibilities, and capacities among institutions on FSM.

### Municipal Capacity Building Needs Assessment for Two ULBs in Odisha by CPR

This study entailed a qualitative survey across a wide range of stakeholders including Angul and Dhenkanal ULBs in Odisha, state officials as well as SBM project monitoring unit (PMU) and technical support unit officials. The stakeholders' capacity was strengthened by organising a master trainers programme and learning visits to deepen their understanding of FSM technologies, O&M and reuse of FSTP by-products. Also, the training modules on non-sewered urban sanitation for Odisha were developed under this project. Capacities of state government stakeholders were built through study visits nationally and globally to understand various policies, legislations and regulations practised by other states and countries on FSM.

Handholding support to two ULBs and the state government was provided by developing case studies on community engagement, supporting plans for the construction of faecal sludge treatment plants in Dhenkanal and Angul towns of Odisha, and O&M plans for sustaining the FSTPs. The experience of Project Nirmal in enhancing the capacities of ULBs like Angul and Dhenkanal has brought rich dividends as these small towns have emerged as pilots for many other pro-poor initiatives in the state.

### Augmenting skills of the city managers: UMC

The CSO, UMC, strives to improve the efficiency and skills of city managers through regular training and capacity-building exercises that enable a better understanding of obstacles and encourage faster solutions. Through its wide network of experts, resource persons and training organisations with adult learning methodologies, it periodically partakes in tailor-made capacity-building plans, study tours and internships to create specific training programmes. Additionally, it also undertakes training needs assessments, designs training tools and recently launched an e-learning portal for city managers.

One of the major innovative interventions of UMC has been anchoring the Performance Assessment System (PAS) for Urban Water Supply and Sanitation, a seven-year action research project, initiated by CEPT University with funding from the Bill and Melinda Gates Foundation in 2009. PAS aims to develop better information on water and sanitation performance at the local level to be used to improve the financial viability, quality and reliability of services. It uses performance indicators and benchmarks on water and sanitation services in all the 400-plus urban areas of Gujarat and Maharashtra.

---

**Box 7.2 Performance Assessment Systems (PAS) for urban water supply and sanitation in Gujarat and Maharashtra**

The PAS for Urban Water Supply and Sanitation project in Gujarat and Maharashtra (2009–14) was sponsored by the Bill and Melinda Gates Foundation. In partnership with the CEPT University, Ahmedabad, UMC implemented this programme in Gujarat.

PAS is aligned with the Service Level Benchmarking (SLB) programme of the MoUD, GOI. It aims to measure, monitor and improve performance assessment of the municipal water supply and sanitation services in urban areas of Gujarat and Maharashtra. Under this programme, UMC is now working with a few ULBs to support improvements in data reliability as well as actual service delivery under the following themes – septage management in non-sewered cities, low-cost wastewater treatment methods, public grievance redressal systems and management information system for improved reliability of data.

The main objectives of the PAS were to (a) develop and implement a performance measurement system for regular and reliable Urban Water Supply and Sanitation (UWSS) information; (b) design and share results with city governments, state government agencies, other stakeholders and various media through a performance monitoring and dissemination system for use in decision-making, providing incentives and influencing demands and (c) facilitate performance improvement plans by the city with support from the state government, NGOs and the private sector.

Further, UMC developed a PAS film in the local language and a framework for performance improvement plans (PIPs)/information system Improvement plan (ISIP) to enable a better understanding of the programme. The same was distributed to ULB staff and other stakeholders at the local level. UMC has documented leading practices followed by ULBs in Gujarat in a catalogue titled, 'What Works'. UMC has also made two films on best practices titled: (i) *Performance Measurement & Improvement* and (ii) *Efficient Water Quality Monitoring*.

*Source*: UMC (2014)

A follow-up of this work was the City Sanitation Plan of Ahmedabad for which the Ahmedabad Municipal Corporation (AMC) appointed UMC in 2011. It encompassed a plan of action for achieving 100 percent sanitation in the city of Ahmedabad through demand generation and awareness campaigns, sustainable technology selection, construction and maintenance of sanitary infrastructure, provision of services, O&M issues, institutional roles and responsibilities, public education, community and individual action, regulation and legislation.

These interventions were then proposed to be scaled up in form of policy through the Ahmedabad Sanitation Action Lab (ASAL), supported by the USAID, for implementing innovative solutions to school sanitation and sanitation problems in informal settlements and slum-like settlements of Ahmedabad, in coordination with the government, NGOs and corporate partners. Through ASAL, AMC has been working on sanitation index, design guidelines for school sanitation and e-courses for city managers on sanitation under SBM. ASAL has aligned its activities with SBM and the Mahatma Gandhi Swachhta Mission of the State Government of Gujarat.

UMC is a pioneer in training and capacity building of city managers and uses various tools, including online courses under SBM. UMC is currently handling the end-to-end development of 85 tutorials, including content development, moderation and a digital resource library. It actively uses movies, documentaries, street theatre, books, newsletters and flashcards as dissemination tools. UMC has also bridged academia with urban management and is one of the key anchors of the Habitat Management Course at CEPT University.

### A key resource centre for capacitating key stakeholders: Gramalaya

Gramalaya is an approved key resource centre with the Ministry of Drinking Water and Sanitation, GOI. It has been an active partner of the authorities concerned in declaring more than 187 informal settlements in Trichy City (Tamil Nadu) as open defecation free (ODF). It played an instrumental role in facilitating Tiruchirappalli City Corporation to come out as the sixth cleanest city in India and the first such city in Tamil Nadu.

Gramalaya's involvement resulted in the alteration of dry earth latrines into modern flush toilets and the eradication of manual scavenging in the city of Tiruchirappalli. Across the jurisdiction of Tiruchirappalli City Corporation, 126 informal settlement communities maintain sanitary complexes under the pay-and-use system. An important outcome of the social innovation that was set in motion by Gramalaya's work in urban sanitation was bringing in women as important stakeholder in the project. Gramalaya by handed over the toilets to women self-help groups (SHGs) for operation and maintenance after the construction or refurbishment of community toilets by the city corporation. This had a ripple effect by generating confidence among women and bringing them into decision-making roles on other issues of slum welfare as well. The corporation endorsed the groups for running the community-managed pay-and-use toilet systems. It demonstrated that community involvement and adequate handholding in the maintenance of community toilets are viable options that can be successfully replicated elsewhere. Furthermore, earning from user charges could be a good revenue model for informal settlement communities with a sustainable approach.

---

**Box 7.3 National Institute of Water and Sanitation (NIWAS)**

Has established the National Institute of Water and Sanitation (NIWAS) with its intervention spanning over 20 years of work in the rural, urban and coastal areas (tsunami-affected fishing villages) reflecting on the key innovations like child-friendly toilets, community-managed pay-and-use toilet systems, school health intervention, toilet technology park, the introduction of water saving baby pans and toilet pans for rural areas.

As part of NIWAS, Gramalaya has been offering training on water and sanitation as well as community development to government officials and local community-based organisations working in rural and urban areas. Stakeholders are capacitated as master trainers, facilitators, volunteers and peer educators to serve the promotion of water and sanitation. The capacity-building training is regularly revised on the basis of feedback from the trainees about the relevance of training content and methodology. The training centre also provides training and capacity-building support to schoolteachers, mid-meal workers, masons and *panchayat* presidents.

*Source*: Gramalaya (n.d.b)

---

### Collaborative initiatives: SCBP of the NIUA

Sanitation Capacity-Building Platform (SCBP) is a learning coalition anchored by NIUA and works as a collaborative initiative of experts and organisations committed to supporting and building the capacity of ULBs, national nodal training institutions, academia and the private sector to plan, design and implement decentralised sanitation solutions. The platform lends support to MoHUA, GOI, by focusing on urban sanitation and supports states and cities to move beyond their ODF status by addressing the safe disposal and treatment of human faeces.

The platform promotes non-networked sanitation systems and has been operational since 2016. Over the years, SCBP has developed as a credible platform with 20 partners of the National Faecal Sludge and Septage Management Alliance (NFSSMA), eight nodal national training institutes and nine university partners. Together this platform has developed a portfolio of standardised FSSM training modules, policy papers, technical reports and research reports.

The SCBP portal is a knowledge platform on decentralised urban sanitation. With an overload of information on the net, this site provides a resource centre for learning and advocacy material, important government orders and reports, training modules, workshop reports and publications produced under SCBP. It also shares the most relevant work on decentralised sanitation from other organisations including reports, publications, videos and learning material.

### *Innovation in participatory learning for elected councillors: PRIA*

PRIA has been known for its innovative participatory learning methodology for developing the capacities of development professionals. It has developed an innovative pedagogy for training on waste management based on a deeper analysis of the roles, responsibilities and aspirations of elected councillors, as understood through the continuous engagement with them over the years. A thorough understanding of learners pointed out a vast variety of socio-demography (age, gender and literacy levels), occupations, priorities and choices. The focus areas of the participatory training were determined after knowing the background of the learners (elected councillors), which aimed to build knowledge and awareness rather than skills.

The learning methods were selected based on the focus areas of training, which covered methods like learning games, case studies, small group discussions and brief lectures (deliberations). Learning games were designed as fun games to facilitate the learning of complex terminologies through picture cards and diagrams. The first set of learning games focused on de-jargonising terminologies contextual to waste management. The participants were observed to enjoy this as they could visualise the terminology through the picture drawn on the back of the card and matched the terminology cards with the picture cards. The facilitator helped them to understand the terminologies through a debriefing session. Another game included a cut–paste and draw activity to explain the flow of liquid waste (black water) in the city. The participants took great interest in first sticking shapes and later connecting them through red and green colours to show the flow and quantity of liquid waste generated and disposal practices prevailing in their respective cities. These games created a clear appreciation of the situation in the respective cities, which was aligned with the prevailing or upcoming planning or implementation interventions being undertaken by the executive wings of the ULBs.

The small group discussions around issues related to liquid waste management were designed following the 'adult learning' principles. The session with group discussions attempted to value and nourish the experience of the elected councillors (learners) during the learning process so that they were not threatened by the learning process. In the session, all participants discussed in smaller groups and presented their views on how to enhance citizen engagement in liquid waste management and presented strategies formulated using their own experience and local considerations. An audio-visual case study created a good backdrop for this exercise and exposed learners to good practices elsewhere to enable them to contextualise in their contexts. Small informative lectures on topics like FSSM Policy were supported by real-life examples and leaflets written in an easy-to-understand manner.

## 4. CONCLUSION

Despite the clear recognition that large capacity gaps exist in ULBs, a systematic approach to capacity building of the city system is almost missing in action. There is a dire need to address capacity gaps in ULBs in a holistic manner (Jha, 2018). Improved processes, technologies and innovations need to be integrated significantly towards enhancing the knowledge base and skills of human capital. This has further propelled the need to reimagine the capacity building of ULBs through training-need analysis, database management of quality training materials and organising field-based training.

The innovative capacity-building practices analysed in this chapter demonstrate that with a concerted strategy, a coherent approach and the right investments, the existing capacity gaps can be effectively addressed. The huge task of the ULB capacity enhancement exercise necessitates decentralisation of the delivery effort too. This further underpins the need for a cheaper, decentralised solution that allows capacity-building inputs to be provided through local arrangements in partnership with a local institution. Importantly, training institutions to encompass a wide range of private, academic, governmental and non-governmental organisations will not merely help bridge the shortage of capacity-building institutions but also offer a whole novel perspective to enrich municipal thinking and a greater comprehensiveness in understanding issues and finding solutions.

The social innovations in the capability building of ULBs need to include accountability, performance assessment and monitoring in all the programmes and schemes. Leaving aside the large municipal corporations, the ULBs are scarcely able to set aside adequate resources for training. This underpins the need for the union and state governments, other funding agencies and the larger ULBs themselves to explore all possible ways of identifying resources for experimenting with newer elements of capacity building of ULBs.

Operating with inefficient ULBs would result in inefficient economies, poor living conditions and a nation with unrealised potential. Thus, it is going to take a concentrated effort from the government to put together an innovative municipal capacity-building management system that will envision what cities need for the next decades and invest in a cadre of ably equipped people who will hold these dynamic spaces together and create an overall environment where social innovation in urban sanitation can thrive.

This chapter emphasises the relevance and importance of enhanced capacities of all stakeholders to promote inclusive sanitation in urban areas. Capacitated human resources with equipped material and technical capabilities in ULBs (as they are responsible for delivering sanitation services in the cities) help in furthering social innovations around community engagement, increasing access and usage of affordable services, promoting simple technological solutions, giving adequate attention to monitoring and evaluation systems and improving O&M of the infrastructure created. Scaling up social innovations by CSOs is dependent on two key factors: adequate capacities of ULBs to adopt a city-wide approach for social innovations and greater recognition of social innovations in policy frameworks to achieve the impact at a larger scale. The next chapter on **Urban Sanitation: Policy Research and Advocacy** touches upon the importance of embedding these social innovations in policy frameworks at the State and National levels for a greater impact on the lives of the most marginalised population residing in urban poor settlements across geographies of the county.

## Notes

1 As per the Census 2011 statistics, about 81 percent urban Indian households had access to latrine facilities, while 13 percent urban households practised OD and the remaining 6 percent relied on CTs/PTs. Approximately 626 million people in India practised OD (Source: Joint Monitoring Programme UNICEF-WHO 2012).
2 OSS systems help safely contain the waste from toilets and provide primary treatment in situ, if corrected properly.
3 Deendayal Antyodaya Yojana – National Urban Livelihood Mission (DAY-NULM) aims at universal coverage of the urban poor for skill development and credit facilities. It strives for skills training of the urban poor for market-based jobs and self-employment, facilitating easy access to credit.
4 Prime Minister Awas Yojana (PMAY) is a national flagship programme for affordable housing.
5 Now renamed as the Ministry of Housing and Urban Affairs (MoHUA).

# 8 Urban Sanitation
## Policy Research and Advocacy

## 1. INTRODUCTION

This chapter dwells on the role of policy research, outreach and advocacy in strengthening and scaling up social innovations to address the unmet needs of urban sanitation in India. The instruments of policy research, outreach and advocacy have been used by many civil society organisations (CSOs) that have been studied and are discussed in this chapter. Policy research, analysis, dissemination and knowledge-based advocacy have been important tools that CSOs have used to both inform their community-based social innovation practices and attempt to scale up these innovations in partnership with other CSOs and different tiers of governments. While many CSOs have undertaken policy research and advocacy, the approach to both alongside the thematic priorities has varied considerably. This chapter enquires what have been the prominent policy research and advocacy approaches used by the CSOs and how these different approaches could be understood by each other.

All research studies have a common goal to produce new knowledge and explanations. On the other hand, all innovations need to have a research component, or what is commonly known as research and development (R&D). This chapter presents various cases of research that have produced new knowledge and have often, especially in the case of CSOs involved in social innovation, developed a solution. To that extent, most research studies by CSOs have primarily focused on identifying gaps in policy and policy implementation. This chapter, therefore, focuses on two central questions. First, what kinds of research and knowledge sharing in the urban sanitation sector have contributed to (a) creating enabling conditions for social innovations to take off at the community level and (b) identifying the concurrent issues that allow community-level innovations to be scaled up through public policy? Second, what kinds of research sharing and innovations in advocacy have contributed to these social innovations in urban sanitation becoming impactful at a wider scale?

With this goal in mind, the chapter first reviews the literature on concepts of policy research and advocacy to draw up a framework to locate the efforts

DOI: 10.4324/9781003197102-8

of the social innovation work of CSOs in recent times. Most CSOs have made different contributions to understanding and meeting unmet needs in urban sanitation, while primarily relying on different advocacy tools reflective of their mandates. The second part of the chapter locates these different approaches within the developed framework and discusses the key efforts of CSOs. The final section summarises how these different approaches, coalitions and networks not only remain relevant but also influence policies to meet the shifting goals of urban sanitation in India. In conclusion, it also discusses how these multiple approaches contribute to furthering the understanding of the importance of policy research and advocacy for social innovations to be successful in meeting India's unmet urban sanitation needs.

## 2. A FRAMEWORK FOR POLICY RESEARCH AND ADVOCACY AS A TOOL FOR SOCIAL INNOVATION IN URBAN SANITATION

**Policy Research and Analysis:** Policy research is primarily viewed as an analysis of the social impacts of pre-existing public policies or those of large-scale public sector development projects. Policy research has typically been best conducted by organisations that specialise in research, units that are close to the policymakers (attentive to their problems and aware of their constraints) but are also sufficiently independent to allow critical analysis (Weimer & Vining, 2017). It has been centrally concerned with mapping alternative approaches and with specifying potential differences in the intention, effect and cost of various programmes. Policy research is understood to be more encompassing than direct policy analysis, long term in its perspectives and more concerned with the goals of the social unit for which the policy is crafted. On the other hand, policy analysis has more targeted goals of analysing and developing alternatives to particular policy actions. Policy research is useful for the reality-testing of a system, especially in circumstances when reality leaves the policy assumptions behind. Hence, it helps in the institutionalisation of the responsibility to prepare alternative rationales and to pry the policymaker loose, from her/his antiquated assumptions (Etzioni, 1971).

Policy research itself focuses on understanding social issues in primarily two ways. The first is *policy-relevant* research where the decision to pursue an investigation into the problems raised by policymakers is taken by the researchers themselves; and, therefore, researchers initiate and often control the agenda. The second is *policy-directed* research where the researchers are involved only once the issues have been identified and often addressed by policymakers. In the latter case, the researchers have much less control over the agenda and are focused on understanding the effectiveness of the policy action (Johnston & Plummer, 2005).

While there are no clear defining criteria for conducting policy-relevant research, it is mostly gathered through a set of principles identified in the existing literature and through practice. The set of principles that guides researchers and creates an enabling environment for relevant research to flourish are referred to as 'embeddedness in policy context', 'internal and external validation', 'responding to policy questions and objectives', 'time-liness', 'constructing an analytical and policy perspective', 'openness to change and innovation' and 'realistic about institutional capacity' (Ordóñez & Echt, 2016). Underpinning the aforementioned broad principles, policy-relevant research needs to be meaningful within and outside the organi-sation's view alone and needs to include other stakeholders' perspectives to strengthen the research agenda. Additionally, it should respond to key policy questions and objectives by critically looking at policy problems. It should go beyond the obvious and narrative descriptions of the situation and make sound contributions by embedding policy problems within the research analytical framework. Such analytical frameworks also propose a pragmatic approach to the research design based on the specific policy prob-lem, appropriate method, time limit and institutional capacity (Ordóñez & Echt, 2016). Thus, to support the researchers' and research organisations' efforts in conducting policy-relevant research, the above-mentioned princi-ples can help in setting out a research framework with the tools and process to improve the organisations' influence in the policy debate.

Based on the experience of practitioners and academicians, policy research can be defined as the 'process of researching on, or analysis of, a fundamen-tal social problem to provide policymakers with pragmatic, action-oriented recommendations for alleviating the problem' (Majchrzak, 1984).

**Linking Research Dissemination and Innovations in Advocacy:** When the policy-relevant research is completed and has established the origins and nature of the problem (to some degree of certainty), for policy and social change the concerned stakeholders have to be convinced that the causes have been properly established and understood, an issue that has been at the core of much debate. This requires research outreach, dissemination and advocacy either by the researchers themselves or by those with whom they are linked (Johnston & Plummer, 2005). This way, advocacy becomes a core dimension where researchers may be involved, operating separately from the policymakers (through institutions such as CSOs and the media) to embed and sustain the case for change.

'Policy advocacy thus can be defined as the process of negotiating and mediating a dialogue through which influential networks, opinion leaders and ultimately decision-makers take ownership of your ideas, evidence, and proposals, and subsequently act upon them' (Young & Quinn, 2012). Research-based advocacy is further understood as the strategies and pro-cesses by which CSOs or social movements seek to influence public policy or people's ideas and behaviour to trigger and encourage social change.

Research outreach, dissemination and advocacy approaches can be broadly categorised as (a) those that target policymakers directly (direct route) or (b) those that attempt to build a broad consensus across stakeholders and the population at large so that they would influence policymakers (indirect route). Each of these categories relies on different research outreach, dissemination and advocacy instruments but both benefit from advocacy through coalitions or networks of different CSOs advocating similar issues and approaches.

In a direct advocacy approach, the researchers reach out to disseminate their research findings by directly targeting the policymakers by using instruments, including small, closed-door meetings or round table discussions and technical engagements with the government through committees. Direct communication with decision-makers through private communications from credible experts has also emerged as a powerful advocacy tool (World Health Organization, 2008). On the other hand, the indirect route to policy advocacy reaches out to a wider set of stakeholders and can include public education; open seminars and workshops; influencing public opinion through publishing findings in the media and running campaigns, among others.

Engaging with media to reach the right audiences through public campaigns and generating outreach material is seen as an essential tool for advocacy. This broadly includes a variety of campaigns using techniques such as chain e-mails or letters, opinion pieces and letters to the editor in newspapers, newsletters, celebrity endorsements, media partnerships with newspapers, journalists and filmmakers, web-based bulletins and online discussions, public events and large-scale advertising campaigns. Advocacy can be made more effective through specialised training (GrantCraft, 2005).

While specific actions that form research dissemination and policy advocacy is easily identifiable, the relevance of specific advocacy instruments has escaped critical attention and the impact of each of these instruments differs due to contextual factors. Given that any or any combination of instruments could be relevant, each policy research project is expected to determine its outreach and advocacy plan and activities (Gen & Wright, 2013).

In both these cases, however, creating coalitions and networks of advocates from similar organisations has also been widely practised as an advocacy strategy, to magnify research findings. This approach of building a coalition of interests across stakeholders strengthens organisational capacity and alliances, increases data and analysis from a social justice perspective and supports specific problem definition and solution as well as policy options while giving greater visibility to the issue of concern in policy processes, often resulting in positive policy outcomes (Primo, 2010).

Advocacy, therefore, is seen as a potent tool to advance public debate on pertinent social issues through sustained coalitions among constituency groups, researchers and experts in communications and public policy. Advocacy has thus far emerged as a very relevant instrument for the dissemination of policy research aimed at clarifying public issues, weighing the merits of various options and firming up the case for the solutions that work best.

## 3. CROSS-CUTTING CONTOURS OF POLICY RESEARCH AND ADVOCACY

The practice of policy research and advocacy by organisations has outpaced its theoretical development. Yet the importance of a theoretical grounding for policy research and advocacy campaigns has increased with the need for accountability and an understanding of advocates' contributions to policy development. Increasing complexities, with technical consultations, outsourced project management units, think tanks and CSOs in the policy-making process, have added to the complexity of policymaking. Within this wide variety of institutional approaches to policy research and advocacy, a framework that categorises policy research and the advocacy models at play can provide a powerful theoretical framework to explain approaches that the CSOs studied have adopted in urban sanitation in India. The framework presented in Figure 8.1 has been crafted to discuss the variety of approaches discussed in the following sections.

The subsequent sections also describe how community action and institutional action can be synergised through policy research and advocacy so that, equipped with necessary information and ideas of what is feasible at the community level, it becomes easier for people to demand accountability in the arena of urban sanitation and also scale up the local initiatives. In light of the above, the work of various CSOs in the space of policy research and advocacy has been analysed and discussed along with the characteristics of social innovations – *hybridity*, *intersectionality* and *relationship building* (see Chapter 2).

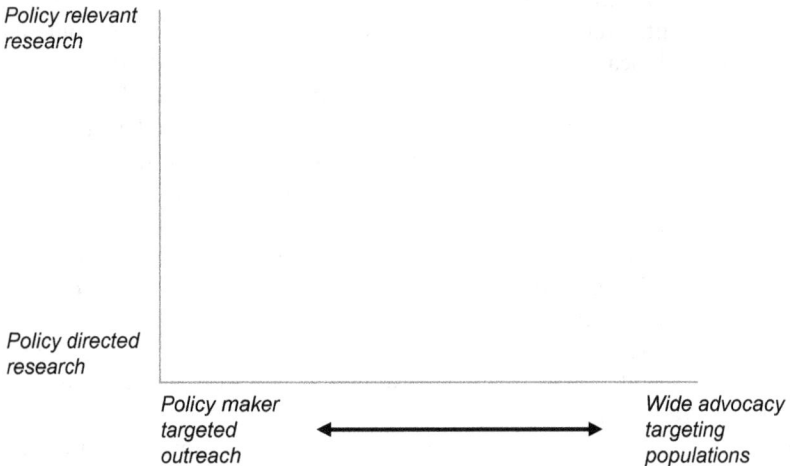

Policy relevant
research

Policy directed
research

Policy maker          Wide advocacy
targeted               targeting
outreach               populations

*Figure 8.1* Conceptual framework for research and advocacy by CSOs. *Source:* Authors

**Policy Research for Alternative Technology Adoption and Mainstreaming:** Research for technology innovation and adoption is an important area of policy research since the efforts to improve sanitation in southern geographies became an international development agenda in the 1970s. While there were some important local innovations in sanitation technologies in the southern countries even before that, a more robust process of innovation and scaling up the use of innovative technologies was put in place as part of an international development agenda that saw improved water and sanitation becoming a core focus area. The research and innovations in water and sanitation technologies were part of a wider search for appropriate technologies across development sectors, which would be more suited for the circumstances in southern countries, including India. The search for alternative water and sanitation technologies was an important part of this area of appropriate technologies. This effort was also strongly influenced, especially in CSO approaches, by the concepts popularised by the influential work of the economist, EF Schumacher (1973). He advocated that the poor countries on the trajectory of ever-increasing growth might realise progress in productivity by adopting advanced but appropriate technologies to the unique needs of each developing country. The appropriate technologies that were developed and propagated, therefore, not only responded to issues such as low-cost systems, use of local materials and skills and the prominence of local maintenance of the built infrastructure but were also associated at great value with the solution being decentralised and at human scale (see Chapter 6 for detailed discussion). This approach was a significant shift from water and sanitation technological approaches adopted in the west since the 1850s, which by the 1970s were considered to be inappropriate, as they were expensive, centralised and based on technologies and technical capacities not available in lower and middle-income countries. By the 1970s, the approach to expand public health infrastructure in the southern countries had gained momentum.

In this section, research efforts by Centre for Science and Environment (CSE), Consortium for DEWATS dissemination (CDD) and Development Alternatives (DA) are discussed and the *intersectionality* between emerging appropriate technologies and diffusion through policy research and advocacy modes are explored. CSE's case study sheds light on how technological solutions need to be socially innovative for them to meet local circumstances of the physical and social context, while mainstreaming lesser appreciated issues, such as water efficiency and conservation, including reuse/recycling of treated wastewater. CDD's technology research and social innovation processes and products (by validating sanitation products on the field, piloting them and scaling them up) have benefitted and contributed to new *relationship building* between previously disjointed individuals and groups have resulted in the diffusion of its ideas and models. Finally, we examine DA's research on green technology innovations for addressing poverty alleviation and economically scalable development outcomes through the adoption of the *hybridity* of multiple distinct elements, such as technologically innovative toilet solutions, advocacy and capacity building of masons.

CSE has been perusing policy research and advocacy across several fields including water and wastewater, habitat, waste, energy recycling, climate change and food and toxins, among others. It has emerged as a key research institution in the country in the water and sanitation space. Much of its technical and policy research has been supported by strong advocacy and outreach. In India, it was among the first institutions that undertook independent policy-relevant research to develop an alternative understanding of environmental and technological issues, especially concerning water and sanitation. Policy-relevant research, such as the continued relevance of traditional water management methods, was brought to the fore in an influential research study entitled, 'Dying Wisdom' (1997), which exposed the modern relevance of traditional water arrangements. Following this, another study on 'Making Water Everybody's Business' (2001) connected the theory and practice of rainwater harvesting (RWH) to methods and suggestions on solutions for planners and policymakers. In sanitation and wastewater management too, the report entitled, Excreta Matters (2013), brought to the fore the massive issues of water pollution from poor sanitation in urban areas. This formative policy-relevant research followed outreach to policymakers and brought the need for decentralised wastewater management to the fore of discussions on wastewater management in India. The research conducted in producing the *Excreta Matters* report also led to the Ministry of Housing and Urban Affairs inviting CSE to be a Centre of Excellence for the ministry and to help it by creating technical guidance notes for local governments on improving on-site sanitation systems for FSM. Thereafter, more recently, CSE has been working with certain state governments and local bodies in the Ganga Basin to develop low-cost FSM systems.

Having used policy-relevant research as a tool to open debates and provide alternative approaches to wastewater management, CSE is currently engaged in policy-directed research in the Ganga Basin cities, especially in small towns with unmet needs about environmental sanitation, to help state governments develop new policies. CSE's approach to urban sanitation has been key in viewing sanitation not as a technical matter alone but as a social participatory issue intrinsically linked with water management. While CSE's work focused on water pollution and rainwater harvesting in the organisation's early years, the innovations it generated was to include wastewater treatment/management and FSM to the sanitation issue and linking them to the overall issues of environmental pollution. Similarly, CSE has led extensive policy-directed research and produced knowledge/advocacy products, including the 'Handbook on Operation and Maintenance of Decentralised Wastewater Treatment System (DWWTs)' (2020), the 'Guidelines for Faecal Sludge and Septage Management in Bihar and Uttar Pradesh' (2018), the report on 'Managing Septage in Cities of Uttar Pradesh' (2019), a scoping paper on 'Development and Validation of Protocol for Testing Faecal

Sludge and Decentralised Wastewater Technologies' (2017) and several other publications.

CSE has also expanded to put in place a fortnightly magazine, *Down to Earth*, as an effective dissemination and advocacy tool for water and sanitation reforms. It has leveraged partnerships with other CSOs, continually advocating the critical issues of urban sanitation through its national and international networks such as the National Faecal Sludge and Septage Management Forum, Sustainable Sanitation Alliance (SuSanA) forum and the Global E-learning Alliance on Faecal Sludge Management Alliance. CSE, the University of Leeds, WEDC Loughborough, EAWAG-SANDEC, WSP-World Bank and Deutsche Gesellschaft für Internationale Zusammenarbeit (GIZ) are further developing tools for the easy production of standardised shit flow diagrams (SFDs) and service delivery context descriptions.

CDD is a network of organisations that works to innovate, demonstrate and disseminate decentralised, nature-based solutions for the conservation, collection, treatment and reuse of water resources and management of sanitation facilities. CDD has benefitted from technical research on decentralised wastewater technology research from various technical research organisations, including Bremen Overseas Research & Development Association (BORDA), a non-governmental organisation from Germany. Over the years, CDD, in support of decentralised technologies, has expanded into policy-directed research related to developing technical guidance on improved design, implementation, operation and maintenance (O&M) of decentralised systems in the domain of wastewater and FSM. This research has also been applied in the field through research and implementation projects emerging from *new relationships* built through networks of organisations, such as SuSanA and the National Faecal Sludge and Septage Management (NFSSMA), which have resulted in the diffusion of its ideas and models.

CDD has mainly focused on policy-directed research, given that its main interest is to develop alternative decentralised wastewater management technologies and facilities. Some of the policy-directed research undertaken in urban sanitation include 'Understanding Characteristics of Faecal Sludge for Treatment', 'Characteristics and Working of Planted Drying Beds', 'Need and Impact of Anaerobic Digestion on Faecal Sludge', 'Operations and Efficacy of Co-composting for Pathogen Reduction and Efficiency of O&M of the Faecal Sludge Treatment Plant (FSTP) at Devanahalli, Karnataka' and 'Study on Closing Nutrient Loop: Evaluation of Co-Composted Faecal Sludge Application in Agriculture'. Much of these works are new and have helped develop improved products and processes in the operation of local governments or other service provision agencies, which have led to advancements and adoption of improved sanitation systems.

DA's green technology innovations for habitat, water, energy and waste management, which deliver basic needs and generate sustainable livelihoods, have reduced poverty and rejuvenated natural ecosystems in the most backward regions of India. In each of these sectors, it has undertaken important policy-relevant research. DA's social innovation in urban sanitation work in the last decade started with a small initiative to build the capacities of masons to construct toilets and facilitate technological innovations related to pre-fabricated toilets with recyclable materials. It documented and analysed good practices in construction with a focus on eco-construction across the country. The knowledge and lessons from its experiences have been compiled into a large number of knowledge products on technologies for waste utilisation in a circular pathway with improved resource efficiency, environmental benefits, reduced carbon footprint and ecosystem conservation.

DA's advocacy and outreach work to generate policy to scale up the influence of the environmental and climate-resilient approaches is centred around the demonstration of policy relevance through capturing best practices, action-based research and creation of partnerships. Such socially innovative practice-to-policy connect helps in analysing challenges and opportunities in specific green sectors, such as agriculture, buildings, renewable energy, water and waste management, etc., leading to the multiplication and scaling up of replicable solutions. DA's policy-directed research and advocacy have led to the increasing adoption of these climate-resilient and energy-efficient models into a larger section of mainstream construction activities.

**Policy Research and Advocacy for the Safety and Dignity of Sanitation Workers:** This section illustrates the relevant research work of organisations like Urban Management Centre (UMC), Safai Karmachari Andolan (SKA) and Participatory Research in Asia (PRIA) under the broader canvas of sanitation workers' safety and dignity. SKA has essentially been an advocacy organisation, which has used research as a tool to bring to the fore vulnerabilities and communicate the concerns of sanitation workers to policymakers. SKA's work largely stems from *intersectionality* cutting across CSOs committed to the rights of Scheduled Castes and other marginalised communities and *safai karmacharis* such as the All India Sweepers Community, the Adar Shila, the Valmiki Samaj and the Solidarity Group for Children against Discrimination and Exclusion across states. Taking the idea of dignity and rehabilitation of those working on manual scavenging also entailed engaging with the media, including direct action like protest marches. PRIA has undertaken some comprehensive studies on the plight of sanitation workers, especially women sanitation workers and their abysmal working conditions, and how it has been neglected in the discussions, at both the state and societal levels. PRIA's work has centrally focused on the empowerment of the excluded through knowledge building, policy advocacy and capacity building by cutting across organisational, sectoral and disciplinary boundaries. This *intersectionality* has been illustrated in the urban sanitation initiatives undertaken from the overall perspective of improving and sustaining sanitation service delivery. While UMC has made laudable contributions in guiding the government and non-government functionaries through its policy-directed research, it has also helped partner government bodies to improve the condition of sanitation workers under their jurisdictions. UMC's innovative approach based on providing a chain of deliverables in the urban sanitation sector echoes *hybridity* by bringing together multiple elements such as situational assessment through performance monitoring, auditing existing facilities, suggesting improvisation in procedures and systems of the sector along with infrastructural improvements, formulating city sanitation plans and advocating best practices through its city links initiative. Similarly, UMC's interventions in urban sanitation exhibit *intersectionality* by engaging with the city, as well as Central and state governments for various urban management aspects, promoting appropriate technological platforms and advocating with innovative media and communication tools such as films, theatres, books and blogs.

**UMC** provides technical assistance and support to national, state and local governments and their associations for implementing programmes that work towards improvement in cities. UMC's approach to urban sanitation is to improve the entire chain of urban management, focusing on sanitation workers in particular. It has documented the occupational environment of sanitation workers and the risks that they face, underpinning the need to ensure safety and humane working condition in all aspects and activities of sanitation.

Through its policy-directed research, UMC has supported governments in collecting information and data from the ground and suggesting improvisation in procedures and systems, supporting the SBM at the central and state levels and capacitating the service provider through urban management courses. UMC has developed advocacy tools for incorporating innovations identified through its ground-level research such as handbooks, ready-reckoners, manuals and video modules on sanitation workers for functionaries at the city, state and national levels. Such knowledge products guide the ULBs to move towards ensuring the safety and dignity of sanitation workers engaged in their respective jurisdictions. Some of UMC's recent relevant research studies and operational manuals are 'Ensuring Safety of Sanitation Workers: A Ready Reckoner for Urban Local Bodies' (Undated), 'Rapid Assessment Report on Health, Safety and Social Security Challenges of Sanitation Workers during the COVID-Pandemic in India' (2020) and the 'Handbook: Training of Sanitation Workers on Use of Personal Protective Equipment – PPEs' (n.d.).

**SKA** has been raising voices against discrimination of sanitation workers by organising, mobilising and campaigning against atrocities, for the discontinuation of dry latrines and their link with the dehumanising occupation of scavenging. SKA played a laudatory role in bringing about legislative changes towards eradicating manual scavenging from India, particularly in the Employment of Manual Scavenging and Construction of Dry Latrines Prohibition Act, 1993.

In 2003, SKA filed a writ petition in the Supreme Court (W.P. (C) 583 of 2003) to force the implementation of the Employment of Manual Scavengers and Construction of Dry Latrines (Prohibition) Act, 1993. A total denial from the state governments about the existence of manual scavenging was followed by partial admission when SKA produced research evidence in terms of photographic evidence to challenge those claims. The presence of 6.76 lakh manual scavengers from over 21 states and UTs was accepted by the Union Ministry for Social Justice and Empowerment in 2002–2003, alongside the admission of the existence of 92 lakh dry latrines.

Apart from its research efforts of documenting the status and concerns of sanitation workers, SKA has advocated its findings by submitting memorandums to the President, Prime Minister, Ministries, statutory bodies and National Advisory Council. SKA has also compiled and submitted its nationwide database of manual sanitation workers across the country. Following that meeting, the Ministry of Social Justice and Empowerment convened the national consultation in January 2011, which resulted in the setting up of four task forces – to review the act, conduct a national survey and revise the rehabilitation package and sanitation solutions. The President of India at the start of the budget session in March 2012 announced the draft of a new bill for the prohibition of manual scavenging. The Government of India passed the new 'Prohibition of Employment as Manual Scavengers and Their Rehabilitation Act 2013' in September 2013 and issued a Government Notification in December 2013. SKA's research and advocacy was key contributor to this.

To raise awareness of the issues faced by sanitation workers across the country, SKA also publishes *Sangharsh* (struggle), a Hindi magazine highlighting issues about safai *karmachari*. SKA closely works in cooperation and partnership with organisations committed to the rights of Dalits and other marginalised communities in general, and *safai karmacharis* in particular. SKA aims to strengthen a diverse national network of individuals and organisations committed to the eradication of manual scavenging. SKA leverages the network of partners such as All India Sweepers Community in West Bengal, The Adar Shila in Uttar Pradesh as well as groups associated with Dalit rights and research, Valmiki Samaj, Solidarity Group for Children against Discrimination and Exclusion in Delhi to create awareness on the eradication of manual scavenging.

**PRIA**, through building knowledge, raising voices and making democracy work realises its vision of a world based on equity, justice, freedom, peace and solidarity. Following the implementation of the SBM, the plight of the sanitation workers, mostly from the Valmiki[1] communities began attracting a lot of policy attention as well as coverage in the public discourse. Their working conditions, irrespective of whether they were working formally or informally, were found to be abysmal with very little or no access to protective gear, medical support, basic labour rights and dignity. The involvement of sanitation workers in the planning, implementation and monitoring of policies and programmes related to sanitation work, or workers, has been felt to be completely absent. The neglect of their voices suppressed them further, rendering them invisible workers and citizens. Unfortunately, the condition of the women sanitation workers did not receive much attention and has been deeply linked to issues like the perpetuation of caste-based vocation, violence and isolation.

PRIA has undertaken a seminal participatory research study, 'Bodies of Accumulation – A Study on Women Sanitation Workers' (2018a), which brought out the intersectionality of caste, gender and informality that cumulatively and additively aggravate the injustice, insecurity and indignity of women sanitation workers. The study reverberated that women sanitation workers were not only subjected to wage disparity or occupational hazards but also subjugated under the established patriarchal attitudes and behaviours in their homes, communities and workplaces. PRIA's work in this arena offers a powerful example of how social knowledge – in this case, the awareness of caste, class and gender fault lines – can impact the way sanitation workers are received, understood and accepted; and in that light, relevant work by PRIA on sanitation workers is further elicited by 'Research Report: Dusting the Dawn – A Study on Women Sanitation Workers in the City Muzaffarpur, Bihar' (2018b) and the paper, 'Lived Realities of Women Sanitation Workers in India – Insights from a Participatory Research Conducted in Three Cities of India' (2019).

**Research and Advocacy for New Service Delivery Solutions:** This subsection reflects upon the policy research work of the think tank, Centre for Policy Research (CPR), under its Scaling City Institutions for India (SCI-FI) research programme; the development organisations, Centre for Urban and Regional Excellence (CURE) and Nidan, in implementing new service delivery models in the urban sanitation space. CPR-SCI-FI has undertaken pioneering policy-relevant research focused on urban environmental sanitation from an alternative service delivery perspective in secondary cities. The initial multidisciplinary, policy-relevant research exposed how past government programmes pursued underground sewerage as the only solution for environmental sanitation. It brought to the fore how the majority of urban India would benefit from alternative solutions like FSM, shifting the needle on national and state policy to support alternative arrangements. It followed up this work with an action research project called Project Nirmal, in partnership with the Bill and Melinda Gates Foundation, Arghyam and Practical Action along with the Odisha State Housing and Urban Development Department and the District Administrations of two towns (Angul and Dhenkanal) in Odisha. This co-produced project was successful in not only building and operationalising the new service delivery models but also demonstrating the effectiveness of the innovative technological model, which incorporated aspects of low-cost, decentralised and inclusive sanitation service delivery solutions that have now been scaled up across Odisha's ULBs. CPR's years of work reverberate *intersectionality* across varied disciplines and sectors, to further social innovation by developing a set of new relationships between individuals and groups, which has resulted in the diffusion of new service delivery ideas on sanitation. This was backed by policy-directed research in Odisha that helped embed the new approaches in state policy, which was scaled up to provide environmental sanitation to all cities in the state. The collaborative effort of CPR, Practical Action and CDD demonstrate low-cost, decentralised, inclusive and sustainable sanitation service delivery solutions – a *hybrid* approach that re-established new *relations* among stakeholders. Such a collaborative partnership demonstrates institutional action planning as well as a community-led advocacy process realised through better integrated institutional and financial arrangements as well as increased private sector participation.

CURE researches new models centring on communities participating in un-thinking, re-imagining, innovating and de-engineering to develop new solutions for particular circumstances. Its work with communities based on policy-directed research and advocacy demonstrates how a community-led approach can be very effective in meeting the challenges of urban sanitation comprehensively and transparently. Finally, Nidan's work on research and new models is based on the cornerstone that recognises access to sanitation to be a basic human right. Nidan's research and piloting projects show how urban slum communities can gain access to toilets through hardware development and by leveraging existing networks of hawkers and vendors. CURE's work on social innovation in urban sanitation focused on a *hybrid* approach through policy-directed research as it entails the synergy of new technological ideas generated by experts with community-based solutions and resources to co-design and co-implement interventions. This work reverberates with *intersectionality* as it cuts across sectoral and disciplinary boundaries of in-house experts – planners, engineers and architects – and members of the community, particularly the urban poor. Its inter-sectoral outreach included experts in information technology (IT) so that smart IT-based solutions can be used for city sanitation planning. Nidan's work also echoes *intersectionality* by bringing together government agencies, networks and communities in informal settlements, schools and *Anganwadis* as well as sanitation service providers in a multi-sectoral manner to break through various development silos and make sanitation a city-wide agenda. How the hawkers and vendors were integrated into India's urban landscape and brought into the sanitation project by harnessing their networks of vendors and hawkers to raise awareness about toilet usage underscored the elements of *relation building*, which formed the centre stage of Nidan's approach in all urban sanitation programmes.

**CPR** initiated the Scaling City Institutions for India (SCI-FI) programme in 2013 that aimed to better understand the 'governance scale' in Indian cities in tandem with 'sector-specific socio-economic scales' for service delivery. CPR-SCI-FI's research in urban sanitation has encompassed both policy-relevant research and policy-directed research. In the early period, when underground sewerage and centralised treatment was the only nationally acknowledged environmental sanitation option, SCI-FI's research into alternative models for sanitation saw a significant amount of policy-relevant research into the ground realities of sanitation in urban India. Other than analysis based on secondary sources like the Census, it also conducted several ground-level primary surveys to identify the importance of focusing on secondary cities and small towns for urban sanitation investments. It also undertook studies based on secondary academic literature including government policies across countries to identify service delivery models to provide environmental sanitation infrastructure in secondary and tier-II/III cities as well as for the urban poor. This was also backed by policy-directed research on the National Urban Sanitation Policy and the Jawaharlal Nehru National Urban Renewal Mission (JnNURM) projects to understand the support that these national programmes have provided to cities to make progress on urban sanitation. Based on the findings of these research projects, CPR-SCI-FI built a policy narrative on the need to legitimise alternative environmental sanitation approaches, especially FSM in India, with a special focus on secondary cities and small towns. The research clearly showed how past policies and programmes on urban sanitation have failed to promote sanitation investments beyond funding underground sewerage systems, which were restricted to only a few large cities in the country. It then undertook numerous research dissemination and advocacy exercises targeted towards building a community of practitioners and building awareness among policymakers through direct meetings and presentations, national-level workshops and opinion articles in newspapers. These efforts bore multiple fruits, be it in terms of state policies or national policies, including the scheme guidance on the SBM (U), the incorporation of funding support for FSM under the flagship Atal Mission for Rejuvenation and Urban Transformation (AMRUT) and the National Faecal Sludge and Septage Management Policy of 2017.

With these learnings from policy research, supported by specific policy-relevant research of on-ground environmental sanitation conditions in secondary cities in Odisha, the Housing and Urban Development Department (HUDD) invited SCI-FI to pilot this alternative sanitation, i.e., FSM models in two small towns in the state. SCI-FI, supported by HUDD, developed a pilot project for two towns identified by the state. HUDD was interested as it was facing numerous challenges in executing underground sewerage projects in Bhubaneswar, Cuttack and Puri, which also had high-cost implications, implying that if underground sewerage would have to be built across the 111 cities in the state it could take at least another 30 years. HUDD was keen to find an appropriate, low-cost and more easily implementable solution for city-wide environmental sanitation. The two small towns chosen were Angul and Dhenkanal. Project Nirmal furthered efforts in improving sanitation access for all households and integration of FSM in the sanitation value chain by enabling institutional and financial arrangements and increased private sector participation. Additionally, the Odisha Urban Sanitation Policy and the Odisha Urban Sanitation Strategy released in late 2016, supported by SCI-FI, laid out the state strategy for sanitation emphasising alternative solutions. This strategy is under active implementation currently and will ensure improved sanitation across Odisha's tier-II and -III towns and cities.

An ethnographic study on culture and urban sanitation by CPR brought forth the issue of caste and sanitation work and how the hierarchy of sub-castes is present within the caste framework. These sub-castes within scheduled castes are placed on the lowest rung of the caste hierarchy and are engaged in the hazardous cleaning of septic tanks and other sanitation systems engaged as manual emptiers. The research findings were shared at the state level with officials, which led to the enumeration of sanitary workers in Angul and Dhenkanal. The survey assessed the residential, occupational and social vulnerabilities of these sanitary workers. As a result, these manual emptiers were linked to other programmes of the state, districts and CSOs. Fifty sanitation workers in Dhenkanal were trained by UMC in partnership with the sector skill council for green jobs and National Safai Karmachari Finance Development Corporation (NSKFDC) on livelihood opportunities. The state government further scaled up this initiative by linking manual emptiers to mechanical desludging work to provide dignity to such workers. The state government developed and notified a scheme called, 'Garima' (pride), for sanitation workers engaged in cleaning septic tanks and sewers.

Enthused by the useful experience, HUDD expanded its ambition and used AMRUT funds to scale up this model in nine other tier-I cities in the state. By 2018, HUDD had gained tremendous experience in FSM and furthered its ambition to cover other 112 cities in the state with FSM programmes. In a further development, which is ongoing at this juncture, based on another pilot that CPR has been undertaking on linking these urban facilities to rural areas, HUDD and the Panchayati Raj Department have issued new guidelines to connect all urban FSTPs with surrounding villages within a radius of 20 km.

CPR-SCI-FI has undertaken numerous policy-relevant studies to identify challenges and has helped address these issues through its implementation support work in Odisha as well as across the country. Some of the relevant studies undertaken in the urban sanitation space include 'A Tale of Two STPs – Case Study of Puri' (2014), 'Faecal Waste Management in Smaller Cities across South Asia: Getting Right the Policy and Practice' (2016), 'Towards a New Research and Policy Paradigm: An Analysis of the Sanitation Situation in Large Dense Villages' (2017), 'Building Regulations for Faecal Sludge Management: Review of Building Regulations From Indian States' (2018), 'Unearthed – Facts of On-Site Sanitation in Urban India' (2018) and 'Beyond 2019: Why Sanitation Policy Needs to Look Past Toilets' (2017). Furthermore, its policy-directed research has helped develop new policies, regulations and business models for FSM. Advocacy goals were initially directed to bring the important stakeholders on board to understand the relevance and utility of the model at the community, city and district levels with strong support from HUDD. Thereafter, advocacy efforts have shifted to promote a better understanding of FSM at the national level and in other states of the country. SCI-FI has continued to rely on tools such as research dissemination workshops, advocacy through direct meetings and presentations, state-level workshops and opinion articles in newspapers.

CURE believes that its core strength lies in its communitarian approach and ability to facilitate processes that empower people to come together, understand and reflect on their problems, articulate their needs and demands, and formulate solutions and take collective decisions and actions to mitigate the problems. It firmly believes in the wisdom of the community for local development planning and design and in building resilient communities and cities.

CURE's research is aimed at precipitating public actions at local levels. CURE has concentrated on producing policy-directed research to open spaces for either direct non-governmental development actions or to elicit local government action and support. Its research has not prioritised policy-relevant research as it has focused on local and community actions on the ground to develop models that can inform wider policy changes. It has quite successfully used this research approach against broader, macro-level policy-relevant research to open out the narratives it has propagated via experimental actions through development projects in water and sanitation. Some of CURE's very pertinent studies and projects in the urban sanitation space are – 'Pani Aur Swacchta Mein Sajhedari (PASS), Baseline Survey, USAID' (2016) – to address water and sanitation issues in informal settlements of Delhi through the implementation of micro plans for sustainable change.

Its locally specific policy-directed action research has typically used a combination of new technological ideas generated by its in-house experts as well as existing community knowledge and experience to generate the technological and social changes necessary for creating alternative models for the delivery of urban sanitation, especially in low-income communities.

Nidan recognised that access to sanitation is a basic human right and started to provide access to toilets for communities from informal settlements. It has been actively working on sanitation issues focusing on hardware tools for providing technological options and decoding the planning and maintenance frameworks for the community. On the hardware component of the intervention, Nidan drew its lessons from its earlier experiences of toilet construction in rural areas, when it had constructed toilets through a UNICEF-supported project in 1999. It discovered that due to the low-cost toilets delivered with low-quality construction materials, the demand for them kept reducing and to achieve open defecation-free (ODF) areas, it was necessary to look beyond the hardware component to the software component by paying equal attention to behavioural change.

Nidan actively contributes to research and knowledge creation in the sanitation sector. It has partnered with technical institutes such as the National Institute of Technology to research appropriate sustainable solutions for sanitation and construction of Leach Pit facilities with greater relevance, particularly in informal settlements. It has also partnered with the Belgium University on water and sanitation issues in Patna, Bihar. Through its sanitation work, Nidan has also been working for the rights of the sanitation workers and abolishing manual scavenging completely by using appropriate technologies for new toilet construction as well as by mobilising and collectivising the workers themselves. Nidan has collaborated on a study on the 'Legacy of Stench – Lives and Struggles of Safai Karmacharis in Patna' (2011) with the support of Water Aid India and Praxis.

At the core of Nidan's innovation is the coming together of the infrastructure of toilet construction for this section of the community with investment in behaviour change and its proactive engagement as a bridge between the community and sanitation service providers. Nidan is also part of the Swachh Bharat Manch, which is a state-level network in Bihar, working on sanitation issues at both urban and rural levels, and with national-level networks such as Freshwater Action Network South Asia (FANSA) and WASH.

## 4. CONCLUSION

The earlier section reviewed the research and advocacy approaches adopted by some CSOs in scaling up social innovations in the urban sanitation programmes they have been recently undertaking. Figure 8.2 shows how some CSOs have focused on policy-relevant research, while most others have focused on policy-directed research. In terms of advocacy too, a mix of strategies is

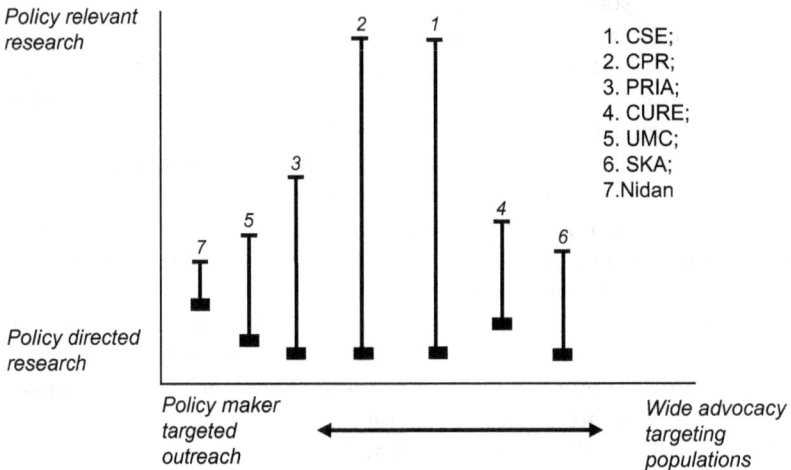

*Figure 8.2* Research and advocacy emphasis by CSOs in urban sanitation. *Source:* Authors

noted between direct policy advocacy and advocacy through constituency building by engaging and targeting wider populations and stakeholders.

For example, SKA's research has been policy-directed where it has resorted to and responded to courts and national policymaking committees to support policy change on issues of sanitation workers. They have been involved in advocacy through building awareness in society at large and the different tiers of government through public campaigns in particular. On the other hand, Nidan, unlike in its programmes related to supporting street vendors, has engaged in site-specific contextual research to help embed social innovations in urban sanitation models, before becoming involved in advocacy by directly approaching and working in a targeted manner with relevant local administrations to scale up these models.

Another comparison of policy research and advocacy is between CSE and CPR's efforts in meeting unmet needs in urban sanitation. CSE and CPR have both perused research studies ranging from policy-relevant to policy-directed research. CPR has adopted a model that relies heavily on policy-relevant research in bringing to the fore the specific geographies that have not been tackled adequately in policy, such as small towns, newly urbanising areas and large, dense villages. CPR has used large databases like those of the Census and National Sample Survey Office (NSSO) to underscore the need to meet unmet sanitation needs. CSE's policy-relevant research on urban sanitation includes the 'Excreta Matters' report, which undertook case studies of more than 70 large and medium towns to bring issues of wastewater management and environmental pollution to the forefront. Both organisations have also been deeply involved recently in perusing the development of FSM models in different geographies, through policy-directed research. CPR has focused on small towns in India, focusing on Odisha under Project Nirmal, while CSE's main geography has been Uttar Pradesh as well as small and medium towns along the Ganga river basin. Both organisations have used direct outreach to policymakers as well as wider advocacy and dissemination targeting wider stakeholders and the population at large. While CSE has used a large number of instruments for wider advocacy through its popular environmental magazine, *Down to Earth*, and public campaigns, CPR has been prolific in the use of opinion pieces in newspapers, digital media and small meetings with relevant stakeholders. In terms of the policy-directed research, on the other hand, both organisations have directly supported the respective state governments in developing strategies and policies for scaling up the urban sanitation models developed in the respective states.

All the CSOs have also demonstrated the value of networks to bring about policy change. This is most strongly demonstrated in the adoption of the National Faecal Sludge and Septage Management Policy, 2017, in numerous state policies and in the incorporation of hybrid toilets in SBM and FSTP funding in AMRUT, which were championed by CSO networks – both national and international – working in the sanitation sector.

These efforts throw light on the centrality of the critical success factors of *hybridity, intersectionality* and *relationship building* for not only creating social innovations in urban sanitation but also ensuring scaling up these models through research and advocacy. These three principles are, therefore, consistent with ensuring the wider involvement of the government to support innovations by scaling them up to cover larger populations with unmet sanitation needs.

In this context, *hybridity*, i.e., the reconfiguration of different pre-existing components is relevant to policymaking too. Both on-ground innovations and research have demonstrated that the creative convergence of different components can create new scaling-up models. An important example from recent times is the dovetailing of different national schemes to address the full chain of sanitation in urban areas. While SBM focused on building safe toilets with containment structures, AMRUT has helped finance the FSTPs to protect the environment from faecal waste pollution. Alongside these programmes, various state government programmes and the national urban livelihoods programme also provided opportunities for self-help groups (SHGs) to engage in sanitation services at scale.

*Intersectionality* has also been important in ensuring that social innovations in a multifaceted challenge like urban sanitation could be scaled up. An example is how the development of slum-upgrading models in some states, low-cost housing programmes and the improvement in piped water services, have contributed to scaling up innovative models. Policy-relevant research from CSOs has also brought to the fore *intersectionality* and the importance of local governments in meeting unmet sanitation needs. It has also exposed the need to focus on environmental pollution management to improve sanitation.

The impact of a social innovation depends on the extent to which it can establish linkages between different sectors, disciplines, organisations and relationships. *Relationship building* among CSOs via networks of organisations, with communities as well as between CSOs and different tiers of the government, has been critical in recognising the social innovations and new, co-developed sanitation models that are being scaled up in India at present.

Policy research and advocacy instruments have been extensively used by the CSOs, as documented in this chapter, to create new knowledge and pursue social innovation. The recent advancement in urban sanitation in India owes a lot to the successful use of these instruments in convincing governments to scale up the social and technological innovations that CSOs have developed. This has been possible in no small measure due to the strong interest that the national government, supported by states and cities, has brought to the sector.

## Note

1 The Valmiki (also Balmik) caste is a Dalit community who have historically experienced sociopolitical as well as economic exclusion, suppression and violence in India. They have been called the 'untouchables' of the caste system.

# Conclusion

This book describes and analyses multifaceted social innovations promoted by several civil society organisations (CSOs) in India to address the gaps in urban sanitation. It demonstrates how these social innovations initially championed by CSOs have over time become part of the next phase of public policies. Social innovations are transformative in nature as they not only find solutions to complex problems but also aim to generate change within the institutional ecosystem responsible for solving those problems by bringing adequate policy focus through action, research, advocacy and strengthening capacities of all stakeholders.

The mapping of sanitation programmes and policies over time in India shows that from independence up until the middle of 2000, rural sanitation received greater attention from policymakers than urban sanitation, with a slew of programmes and schemes by the Government of India (GOI) targeted at villagers to build and use toilets since the 1980s. The challenges of urban sanitation and environmental pollution were not adequately addressed at the national level till the middle of 2000 when the Jawaharlal Nehru National Urban Renewal Mission (JnNURM) was announced. The JnNURM focussed on network sanitation, connecting urban households with sewerage networks in million-plus cities in 2005. Attention to faecal sludge management (FSM) as a sustainable sanitation model emerged only in 2015 in the country, acknowledging the preponderance of onsite sanitation systems in urban India, thereby necessitating an alternative and affordable solution for wastewater treatment. A watershed moment in the policy landscape on urban sanitation came with the launch of the GOI's flagship ambitious programme, SBM, in 2014 and Atal Mission for Rejuvenation and Urban Transformation (AMRUT) in 2015 (both programmes continuing), which focussed on universal access to toilets for the urban poor by offering subsidies and focussing the government's attention on FSM. While the policy landscape was becoming conducive by bringing FSM to the foreground, the unmet needs of the poor to receive affordable services, low-cost infrastructure for improved health outcomes and safety and dignity of sanitation were gaining ground to further spur social innovations.

DOI: 10.4324/9781003197102-9

Other than CSOs, social innovations have been ideated and driven by the government, social entrepreneurs, for-profit organisations and academia as well. However, this book delves into social innovations spearheaded by CSOs who have been actively promoting and facilitating socially innovative models to improve urban sanitation in India. These innovations range from providing low-cost infrastructure solutions, demanding services from the service providers by mobilising citizens, generating awareness to bring changes in attitude and behaviour, building and strengthening community-managed systems for ensuring the sustainability of the created assets, organising informal sanitation workers to demand dignity and justice as well as promote equity and equality, strengthening capacities and building collaboration and partnerships with various stakeholders including the government and undertaking research and advocacy to influence policies for the most marginalised.

Social innovations are local and context-specific, as gleaned through various CSO-led interventions included in this book, but have the potential to disseminate and scale up by receiving policy focus and being diffused to the contexts facing similar intractable challenges and unmet needs. Social innovations need support to thrive and survive. The support they need may include enabling policy, institutions, financing and partnership. In evaluating the role of each of these, we have found the metaphor used by Mulgan et al. (2007) of bees and trees particularly helpful. The bees are the small organisations, individuals and groups who have new ideas and are mobile, quick and able to cross-pollinate. The trees are the big organisations – governments and companies or large NGOs – who may be poor at creativity but are generally good at implementation and have the resilience, roots and scale to make things happen. Both need each other, and most social change comes from the alliances between the two. The CSO case studies discussed in this volume demonstrate similar configurations concerning the relationship with public authorities and programmes.

This unique symbiotic relationship between social innovators and scaling up institutions is exemplified by social innovations in sanitation. Social innovation from the past on twin-pit toilet technology from Sulabh International in the 1970s to eliminate the deplorable, dehumanising and exploitative practice of manual scavenging, pay-and-use toilets by Community Led Total Sanitation (CLTS) Foundation for empowering communities to change their attitude and behaviour to build and use toilets has been reflected in the development of government policies. These novel ideas have been extended to urban areas, hence underscoring the adaptability of social innovations and fostering the symbiotic relationship between bees and trees for innovation to meet unmet needs.

For social innovations to be scalable, they should be based on principles of economic, environmental and social justice. Social innovations are a continuous process as new unmet needs emerge with time. They can help mitigate some intractable problems; but as new challenges emerge, they promote social innovations to grow and adapt to meet the unfulfilled needs of the people. Social innovations need appropriate conditions to take root such as strong leadership and vision by social innovators, partnerships and alliances, enhanced capacities of institutions to respond to intractable problems, empowerment of communities and the most marginalised to gain voices to articulate their unmet needs and demand accountability from the institutions of governance.

This book has attempted to study a set of social innovations in the context of meeting unmet needs in the urban sanitation sector in India. Historically, there is evidence that social innovations in urban sanitation have contributed to the development of solutions that are well accepted by society today. Given the circumstances where public resources were not as significant as they are today in areas of urban infrastructure, including urban sanitation, these past social innovations were easily recognisable and appreciated. Over the last two decades, however, investments in urban sanitation through public finance have been steadily rising across cities in India. With the start of the JnNURM programme, underground sewerage and urban sanitation have become a regular part of all national urban infrastructure investment programmes. With this increasing scale of public finance available for the urban sector, especially in sanitation, the role that social innovations play, especially those anchored by CSOs, has become less visible. Hence, our research has studied recent CSO actions to understand what the role of social innovation by CSOs has been within this changing context.

The book relies on case studies of a set of 15 CSOs to inform its analysis. Using the institutions and the work that they have done as the data to inform the hypothesis, the underlying study that this book covers, CSOs were selected based on certain key themes that have emerged as important tenets in urban sanitation policy and investment. These themes reflect the key areas that are increasingly becoming prominent as some unmet needs have to be fulfilled and include issues around sanitation workers and work conditions; new innovative technologies for sanitation management; behaviour change required in society to adopt new technological innovations and new systems; institutional capacity building – both in public institutions responsible for financing, regulating and implementing urban sanitation programmes and in the wider stakeholder group, which includes community groups, political leadership, research institutions; innovative policy research and advocacy around emerging unmet needs.

Even as urban sanitation improves, new challenges of unmet basic needs for marginalised communities, poor public health and environmental impacts emerge to the fore and become new central needs that the sector has to address. In addition, benchmarks and goals for sanitation have also been changing. Up until 2015 under the international Millennium Development Goals (MDGs) regime, most of the focus internationally was on access to toilets. More recently, however, with the Sustainable Development Goals (SDGs) gathering momentum, the attention has been shifted to the full sanitation value chain of safely managed sanitation, thereby bringing in many new areas for public investment in sanitation programmes. The CSO interventions included in this book demonstrate how they have emerged as key actors working in these futuristic thematic areas.

Each chapter of the book has explored unmet needs for a progressive and sustainable urban sanitation sector and looked at the CSOs who have worked in meeting specific unmet needs. This is important because through their work they have contributed to and influenced the development of past policies, and this space for social innovation by CSOs must be strengthened for future policy on urban sanitation.

## 1. KEY FINDINGS

This book has drawn attention to recent innovative practices in urban sanitation that citizens have initiated, catalysed by CSOs to meet their unmet needs when the institution of the state and the mechanics of the market have fallen short of fulfilling their requirements. Our primary finding has been that it is the CSOs that have helped empower marginalised communities to access urban sanitation services, provided institutional frameworks for solidarity to accompany technical innovation, transformed social relations and encouraged new forms of governance and community participation.

Amid a pandemic that threatens to further widen existing social and economic inequalities, it is imperative to think of social innovations in urban sanitation that gives voice and power to marginalised communities. It is in this context that the multifaceted experiments in urban sanitation undertaken by the host of organisations studied in this book assume significance, as they have all directly or indirectly helped to mobilise the hitherto unorganised community to meet the unmet needs of sanitation. These CSO initiatives have generated a spirit of partnership by facilitating channels of communication between the privileged and non-privileged citizens, creating democratic and participatory forums, investing in the leadership of the poor and vulnerable, connecting government and other stakeholders to create intersectionality in organisation building and making government institutions accountable, among others. It is the CSOs who have recognised that unless the unorganised community is actively drawn into the plan of action, social innovations in urban sanitation will not touch the lives of the very people who need it the most.

The learning that has emerged from the overall research on the urban sanitation landscape in India indicates that CSOs have helped to meet new social needs in newer ways. In meeting unmet needs in urban sanitation in India, the focus has to be both on the vulnerable community and groups who have to be drawn into the ambit of the urban sanitation cover as well as on the conditions of those who provide these services. This includes the sanitation workers and those engaged in the still prevalent practice of manual scavenging, which continues to take place, carrying inescapable associations with the caste system. While the government schemes have now acknowledged the reality of the condition of manual scavenging, the transformative social movement has raised a new public consciousness around sanitation work and the rights and dignity of sanitation workers, including the women in that workforce, and helped forge new solidarities from civil society movements.

A key finding in our study has been that when CSOs work to ensure that appropriate technologies are linked with specific needs of the community – in this case, the sanitation needs of the urban poor and other marginalised groups – the impact of that technology is multiplied. When a mutually reinforcing relationship is established between technological innovation and social needs, the former is much more likely to be accepted and diffused; and to that extent, its full potential is realised. India has learnt – the hard way – that a market-based approach to constructing toilets using the available technology does not solve the urban sanitation problem in its totality. A new thought that links urban sanitation with technology that is not just eco-friendly but also culture-friendly, cost-effective and based on a participatory model is that it will carry with it the possibility of scaling up, without which the urban sanitation problem cannot be resolved. CSOs with their histories of working with participatory models are best equipped to do this.

We found that social innovations in urban sanitation have had the greatest impact where CSOs have invested in building capacities of low-income communities and municipalities to engage in participatory planning and developed the capacities of municipal officials, elected councillors and engineers on key elements of urban sanitation, such as septage management, solid waste management, decentralised water treatment and water sensitive urban design. This is because municipalities have been given the responsibility of implementing programmes of urban sanitation by the government, yet their capacities for carrying this out have not been planned. This is where we have found the role of CSOs, with their rich experience of providing participatory training, playing a critical role. We also found that capacity-building interventions are most effective in bringing transformations at the city level when an ecosystem approach is adopted by addressing the differential learning needs of various actors.

A leitmotif that runs through this entire book is that of behaviour change. This follows from the recognition that unless there is individual and social behaviour change, the best schemes and technologies will not be successful in reaching the goal of sanitation for all. Integral to the process of social innovation is behaviour change of all stakeholders as they interact and engage in a mutual process of co-learning. The organisations carrying out social innovations, the policymakers and the targeted primary stakeholders in the community undergo changes that sometimes occur more noticeably and sometimes in a more subtle manner. Behaviour change is sometimes actively facilitated by a process of strategic communication, which involves applying the processes, strategies and principles of communication to reach out to people with the intent to influence attitudes and bring about positive social change. The case studies we have drawn upon have indicated several such instances when social innovation in urban sanitation tried to consciously bring about this change of attitude and behaviour either through campaign messaging, or the use of mass media and interpersonal messages directed at the urban poor. The mapping of urban sanitation initiatives across the country, which has been the heart of this study, has indicated that several factors influence social and behaviour change. These include knowledge, attitude, people's confidence to practice a behaviour as well as social norms, access, affordability, quality of services and socio-economic factors outside of the family. All these factors have to be taken into account while designing an effective communication strategy for behaviour change.

Behaviour change in urban sanitation is aimed not just at encouraging the community to construct and use toilets but to embrace the complete sanitation value chain. It is also directed at government agencies to encourage thinking across developmental silos and acknowledge that urban sanitation is not just an issue for the municipality or urban development departments in the government, but linked closely to health, social work, education and livelihoods.

Ongoing research and advocacy on urban sanitation create the ambience for social innovations in this arena by synergising community action with institutional action and public policy. Scaling up social innovations may require launching campaigns, research sharing and advocacy in a way that local stakeholders are enthused by the idea of participation in this process. Evidence from multiple case studies suggests that CSOs involved in practice-based research are best equipped to carry out this work, since they are linked to both the community and the institutions.

## 2. NEW FRONTIERS OF SOCIAL INNOVATION IN URBAN SANITATION

This book provides evidence and discusses the continued relevance of social innovation in urban sanitation to meet the unmet sanitation needs in India. It has also discussed and analysed how urban sanitation needs are an evolving process. It discusses how norms of contemporary urban sanitation have progressively become more encompassing across society at large. The SDGs have also significantly changed the aspirational standards from access to basic sanitation to safely managed sanitation. This is also reflected in the GOI's policy progression from Swachh Bharat Mission to Swachh Bharat Swachh Bharat Mission 2.0. Within this context, it is important to keep in mind that even if the SDG targets are met or Swachh Bharat Mission 2.0 is implemented successfully, the unmet needs in urban sanitation will continue to emerge. These unmet needs will not be the same as the ones that have been addressed in the recent past and are being addressed currently but will be a new set of social and environmental concerns related to urban sanitation that will come to the fore. For example, urban sanitation systems as implemented in most parts of the world remain to be highly energy intensive and demand significant resources and in the past have had significant costs to the environment. In the current era of re-evaluating public policies and social lifestyles, based on conservation of energy, reducing greenhouse gases and carbon footprints, it is not hard to imagine that the urban sanitation systems that we are even putting in place today may need further upgradation to respond to the causes that accelerate global warming and other climate change-related challenges.

Another example of a direction where unmet needs could be felt more strongly is in the connection between the levels of services in urban, peri-urban and rural areas in developing countries. While many parts of these urban areas have much higher levels of service today, most of the rural and peri-urban areas have much lower levels of service. As the global population rises, density increases and the demands for universal service levels increase, the challenges of having high levels of services in these areas would also be rising.

These new frontiers of urban sanitation might need to be addressed tomorrow. The continuation of the emergence of new frontiers will lead to new unmet needs in the urban sanitation sector in the future, thereby necessitating further social innovations by CSOs.

# References

Anadon, L. D., Chan, G., Harley, A. G., Matus, K., Moon, S., Murthy, S. L., & Clark , W. C. (2016). Making technological innovation work for sustainable development. *Proceedings of the National Academy of Sciences*, 113(35), 9682–9690. https://doi.org/10.1073/pnas.1525004113.

Backward Classes Commission. (1955). *Report of the backward classes commission* (Vol. I). Government of India. Retrieved from https://dspace.gipe.ac.in/xmlui/handle/10973/33678.

Bandura, A. (1997). *Self-efficacy: The exercise of control*. W H Freeman/Times Books/ Henry Holt & Co.

Barroso, M. J. (2011). Europe leading social innovation. Press release by Social innovation Europe Initiative, Brussels. Retrieved from https://ec.europa.eu/commission/presscorner/detail/en/SPEECH_11_190.

Basu, S. K. (1991). *Report of the Task Force for tackling the problems of scavengers and suggesting measures to abolish scavenging with particular emphasis on their rehabilitation*. Planning Commission, Government of India.

Bauman, Z. (1998). *Culture as Praxis* (2nd ed.). Retrieved from https://uk.sagepub.com/en-gb/eur/culture-as-praxis/book205973

Becker, M. H. (1974). *The health belief model and personal health behavior*. Slack Incorporated©.

Bessette, G., & Rajasunderam, C. (Eds.). (1996). *Participatory development communication: A West African agenda*. International Development Research Centre.

Black, M., & Fawcett, B. (2008). *The last taboo: Opening the door on the global sanitation crisis*. Earthscan.

Cadiz, M. C. (1994). *Communication and participatory development: A review of concepts, approaches, and lessons* (16th ed.). University of the Philippines. https://www.ukdr.uplb.edu.ph/books/16.

Cajaiba-Santana, G. (2014). Social innovation: Moving the field forward. A conceptual framework. *Technological Forecasting and Social Change*, 82, 42–51.

Census. (1981). Government of India. Retrieved from https://censusindia.gov.in/nada/index.php/catalog/28122/download/31304/49962_1981_POR.pdf.

Census. (2011). Government of India. Retrieved from https://censusindia.gov.in/2011-common/censusdata2011.html.

Central Pollution Control Board. (2021). *National inventory of sewage treatment plants*. Ministry of Environment, Forest and Climate Change, GoI. Retrieved from https://cpcb.nic.in/openpdffile.php?id=UmVwb3J0RmlsZXMvMTIyOF8 xNjE1MTk2MzIyX21lZGlhcGhvdG85NTY0LnBkZg==

Chambers, K. K. (2008). *Handbook on community led total sanitation*. Plan International (UK) & Institute of Development Studies (Sussex, UK).

Chaplin, S. E. (1999). *Cities, sewers and poverty: India's politics of sanitation*. SAGE. Retrieved from https://journals.sagepub.com/doi/10.1177/095624789901100123

Chaplin, S. E. (2011). *The politics of sanitation in India: Cities, services, and the state*. S. Bhattarcharya & N. Brimnes (Eds.). Orient Blackswan Private Limited. Retrieved from https://books.google.co.in/books?id=4S4OMwEACAAJ&hl=en

Chaplin, S. E. (2017). *Gender and urban sanitation inequalities in everyday lives: A literature review and annotated bibliography*. Centre for Policy Research. Retrieved from https://www.researchgate.net/publication/324006521_Gender _urban_sanitation_inequalities_and_everyday_lives_A_literature_review_and _annotated_bibliography/link/5ab894c7aca2722b97cf9fc9/download.

Chintan. (2021). *Chintan*. Retrieved from chintan: https://www.chintan-india.org/ index.php/what-we-do

Coffman, J. (2002). *Public communication campaign evaluation: An environmental scan of challenges, criticisms, practice and opportunities*. Harvard Family Research Project. Retrieved from https://archive.globalfrp.org/content/download /1116/48621/file/pcce.pdf.

Consortium for DEWATS Dissemination Society (CDD). (2018). *Compendium of innovative technologies for urban sanitation*, December 2018. Accessed on 2 October 2011. Retrieved from https://www.susana.org/_resources/documents/ default/3-4094-226-1617025910.pdf.

Cornwall, A. (2000). *Sida studies no. 2*. Retrieved from https://cdn.sida.se/ publications/files/sida982en-beneficiary-consumer-citizen---perspectives-on -participation-for-poverty-reduction.pdf

Central Pollution Control Board (CPCB). (2019). *Annual report 2018–19*. CPCB, Ministry of Environment, Forest & Climate Change, Government of India. Retrieved from https://cpcb.nic.in/openpdffile.php?id=UmVwb3J0RmlsZXMvMTExOV8xNTk3MDM3NTM0X21lZGlhcGhvdG.

Craig, G., & Mayo, M. (1995). *Community participation and empowerment: The human face of structural adjustment or tools for democratic transformation?* Zed Books.

Centre for Science and Environment (CSE). (2014). *Decentralised wastewater treatment and reuse: Case studies of implementation on different scale – Community, institutional and individual building*. Retrieved from https:// citeseerx.ist.psu.edu/viewdoc/download?doi=10.1.1.440.2310&rep=rep1&type =pdf.

CSE. (n.d.). *Anil Agarwal environment training institute*. Accessed on 2 October 2022. Retrieved from https://www.cseindia.org/page/aaeti.

Cunha, J., Benneworth, P., & Oliveira, P. (2015). Social entrepreneurship and social innovation: A conceptual distinction. In L. M. Farinha, J. Carmo, J. M. Ferreira, H. L. Smith & S. Bagchi-Sen (Eds.), *Handbook of research on global competitive advantage through innovation and entrepreneurship*. IGI Global, 616–639.

CURE. (n.d.b). *SANMAN: A tool for city sanitation management*. Accessed on 12 September 2022. Retrieved from https://cureindia.org/page35.html.

Dak, T. M. (2007). *Impact of scheme of training and rehabilitation on socioeconomic improvement of scavengers in Rajasthan*. Institute of Social Development.

Retrieved from https://www.niti.gov.in/planningcommission.gov.in/docs/reports /sereport/ser/ser_istr.pdf.

Dalit Network Netherlands. (2013). *Knock the door campaign.* Retrieved from Dalit Network Netherlands http://www.dalits.nl/130812e.html.

Dasgupta, S., Singh, T. and Dwivedi, A. (2020). *Invisible sanitation workers @ Covid 19 lockdown: Voices from 10 cities.* Centre for Policy Research. Retrieved from https://cprindia.org/wp-content/uploads/2021/12/Invisible-Sanitation -Workers-@-Covid-19-Lockdown_Voices-From-10-Cities.pdf

Down to Earth. (2019). *Jal Shakti Abhiyan: What can make it more impactful.* Retrieved from https://www.downtoearth.org.in/blog/water/jal-shakti-abhiyan -what-can-make-it-more-impactful-66878.

Drucker, P. F. (1986). *Innovation and entrepreneurship: Practice and principles.* Harper & Row.

D'Sourza, P. (2016). Clean India, unclean Indians beyond the bhim yatra. *Journal name comes here]* 51(26–27). Retrieved from https://www.epw.in/journal /2016/26-27/commentary/clean-india-unclean-indians-beyond-bhim-yatra .html.

Etzioni, A. (1971). Policy research: The American sociologist. *American Sociological Association,* 6(Supplementary Issue) (Jun., 1971), 8–12. Retrieved from https://www.jstor.org/stable/pdf/27701831.pdf?casa_token=WH-eY _6lYKMAAAAA:AXafVFQoiH_lV6qH1a86_ULsr61JMnrgV4Wk1UruXQbq LJomXBz_j-

Freire, P. (1970). *Pedagogy of the oppressed* (30th anniversary ed.). M. B. Ramos (Trans.). The Continuum International Publishing Group Ltd.

Gen, S., & Wright, A. C. (2013). Policy advocacy organizations: A framework linking theory and practice. *Journal of Policy Practice, 12*(3), 163–193. https:// doi.org/10.1080/15588742.2013.795477

Godin, B. (2012). Social innovation: Utopias of innovation from c.1830 to the present. *Project on the intellectual history.* Working paper no. 11. Retrieved from http://www.csiic.ca/PDF/SocialInnovation_2012.pdf.

Gramalaya. (n.d.a). *Eco-san toilets.* Accessed on 15 September 2022. Retrieved from https://gramalaya.org/eco-san-toilets.

Gramalaya. (n.d.b). *NIWAS resource centre.* Accessed on 15 September 2022. Retrieved from https://gramalaya.org/service/niwas-resource-centre.

GrantCraft. (2005). *The tools of advocacy.* Retrieved from Candid https://grantcraft .org/content/takeaways/the-tools-of-advocacy.

Hall, B., Gillette, A., & Tandon, R. (Eds.). (1982). *Creating knowledge: A monopoly?* Participatory Research Network Series No. 1, PRIA.

Hall, J., Matos, S., & Martin, M. (2014). *Innovation pathways at the base of the pyramid: Establishing technological legitimacy through social attributes.* Retrieved from https://www.researchgate.net/publication/260009638_ Innovation_pathways_at_the_Base_of_the_Pyramid_Establishing_technological _legitimacy_through_social_attributes.

Hellstrom, T. (2004). *Innovation as social action.* https://doi.org/10.1177 /1350508404046454

Hochbaum, G. M. (1958). *Public participation in medical screening programs: A socio-psychological study.* U.S. Department of Health, Education, and Welfare, Public Health Service, Bureau of State Services, Division of Special Health Services, Tuberculosis Program.

International Labour Organization – ILO. (2014). *Resource handbook for ending manual scavenging*. ILO India. Retrieved from http://www.dalits.nl/pdf/Resourc eHandbookForEndingManualScavenging.pdf.

Jayaweera, N. (1987). *Rethinking development communication: A holistic view*. N. J. Amunugama (Ed.). The Asian Mass Communication Research and Information Centre.

Jha, R. (2018). *It is time to reimagine capacity building of ULBs*. Observer Research Foundation. Retrieved from https://www.orfonline.org/expert-speak/it-is-time-to -reimagine-capacity-building-of-ulbs.

Johnston, R. & Plummer, P. (2005). What is policy-oriented research? *Environment and Planning A*. 37, 1521–1526. 10.1068/a3845. Retrieved from https://www .researchgate.net/publication/23539583_What_is_policy-oriented_research.

Lapierre, J. W. (1968). *Essai sur le fondement du pouvoir politique [Essay on the foundation of politics]*. Aix-en-Provence, Ophrys.

Lüthi, C. (2010). Community-based approaches for addressing the urban sanitation challenges. *International Journal of Urban Sustainable Development*, 1(1–2), 49–63. https://doi.org/10.1080/19463131003654764

Majchrzak, A. (1984). *The nature of policy research*. Sage. https://doi.org/10.4135 /9781412985024.n1.

Manyozo, L. (2006). Manifesto for development communication: Nora C. Quebral and the Los Banos School of Development Communication. *Asian Journal of Communication*, 16(1), 79–99. https://doi.org/10.1080/01292980500467632

McNeill, J. (2012). Through Schumpeter: Public policy, social innovation and social entrepreneurship. *The International Journal of Sustainability Policy and Practice*, 8(1), 81–94.

Mendoza, R. U., & Thelen, N. (2008). Innovations to make markets more inclusive for the poor. https://doi.org/10.1111/j.1467-7679.2008.00417.x

Ministry of Housing Urban Affairs (MoHUA). (2021). *Ensuring safety of sanitation workers: A ready reckoner for urban local bodies*. MoHUA, Government of India. Retrieved from https://umcasia.org/what-we-do/ready-reckoner-for-sanitation -workers-safety.

Ministry of Law and Justice. (2020). *The constitution of India*. Legislative Department, Ministry of Law and Justice, Government of India. Retrieved from https://legislative.gov.in/sites/default/files/COI_1.pdf.

Ministry of Urban Development (MoUD). (2008). *National urban sanitation policy*. MoUD, Government of India. Retrieved from http://mohua.gov.in/upload/ uploadfiles/files/NUSP_0.pdf.

Mulgan, G. (2006). The process of social innovation. *Innovation: Technology, Governance, Globalization*, 1(2), 145–162. https://doi.org/10.1162/itgg.2006.1 .2.145.

Mulgan, G., Tucker, S., Ali, R., & Sanders, B. (2007). *Social innovation: What it is, why it matters and how it can be accelerated*. Working Paper. The Young Foundation. Retrieved from https://youngfoundation.org/wp-content/uploads /2012/10/Social-Innovation-what-it-is-why-it-matters-how-it-can-be-accelerated -March-2007.pdf.

Murray, R., Caulier-Grice, J., & Mulgan, G. (2010). *The open book of social innovation*. The Young Foundation. Retrieved from https://youngfoundation.org /wp-content/uploads/2012/10/The-Open-Book-of-Social-Innovationg.pdf.

Mutekwe, E. (2012). The impact of technology on social change: A sociological perspective. *Journal of Research in Peace, Gender and Development*, 2(11), 226–238. Retrieved from http://www.interesjournals.org/JRPGD.

Nair, P., & Dwivedi, A. (2017). *Capacity building need assessment of cities (Angul and Dhenkanal) and state government on sanitation: A case of Odisha.* Centre for Policy Research (CPR). Retrieved from https://www.cprindia.org/research/reports/capacity-building-need-assess.

National Institute of Urban Affairs – NIUA. (2021). *Understanding effectiveness of capacity development: Lessons from sanitation capacity building platform (SCBP).* NIUA. Retrieved from https://niua.org/intranet/sites/default/files/1506.pdf.

National Master Plan – IDWSSD. (1983). *National master plan India: International drinking water supply and sanitation decade 1981–1990.* Ministry of Works and Housing, Government of India. Retrieved from https://www.ircwash.org/sites/default/files/822-IN83-2473.pdf.

NSKFDC. (n.d.). The self employment scheme for rehabilitation of manual scavengers (SRMS). Accessed on 15 September 2022. Retrieved from https://nskfdc.nic.in/en/content/revised-srms/self-employment-scheme-rehabilitation-manual-scavengers-srms.

National Sample Survey Organisation (NSSO). (1998). Drinking Water, sanitation and hygiene in India, NSS 54th Round (January–June 1998). Ministry of Statistics and Programme Implementation, Government of India. Retrieved from http://www.icssrdataservice.in/datarepository/index.php/catalog/54/download/664.

Neyere, J. K. (1973). *Freedom and development.* Oxford University Press.

NFSSM Alliance, & NITI Aayog. (2021). *Faecal sludge and septage management in urban areas: Service and business models.* Retrieved from https://niti.gov.in/sites/default/files/2021-01/NITI-NFSSM-Alliance-Report-for-digital.pdf.

Ngigi, S., & Busolo, D. N. (2018, September). Behaviour change communication in health. *International Journal of Innovative Research and Development*, 7(9). https://doi.org/10.24940/ijird/2018/v7/i9/SEP18027

Nidan and Praxis. (2011). A legacy of Stench! An account of lives and struggles of Safai Karmacharis in Patna. Retrieved from https://www.praxisindia.org/_files/ugd/8a8dda_743c24bdc2e64e6488f599ae095a8c09.pdf.

Nisbet, E. K., & Gick, M. L. (2008). Can health psychology help the planet? Applying theory and models of health behaviour to environmental actions. *Canadian Psychology/Psychologie Canadienne*, 49(4), 296–303. https://doi.org/10.1037/a0013277.

Nussbaum, M., & Sen, A. (1993). *The quality of life.* Clarendon Press.

Ogburn, W. (1964). *Culture and social change.* University of Chicago Press.

Ordóñez, A., & Echt, L. (2016). *What are the principles of policy relevant research?* On Think Tanks. Retrieved from: https://onthinktanks.org/articles/what-are-the-principles-of-policy-relevant-research.

Participatory Research in Asia (PRIA). (2018a). *Bodies of accumulation: A study on women sanitation workers.* PRIA. Retrieved from https://www.pria.org/knowledge_resource/1554111089_Research%20Report-%20Bodies%20of%20Accumulation-%20A%20Study%20on%20Women%20Sanitation%20Workers%20in%20Jhansi.pdf.

PRIA. (2018b). *Dusting the dawn: A study on women sanitation workers in the city Muzaffarpur, Bihar*. PRIA. Retrieved from https://www.pria.org/knowledge_resource/1554103696_Research%20Report-Dusting%20the%20Dawn-A%20Study%20on%20Women%20Sanitation%20Workers%20in%20the%20City%20Muzaffarpur-Bihar.pdf.

PRIA. (2019). *Lived realities of women sanitation workers in India insights from a participatory research conducted in three*. PRIA. Retrieved from https://pria.org/knowledge_resource/1560777260_Occasional%20Paper%204%20(2019)%20(Lived%20Realities%20of%20Women%20Sanitation%20Workers%20i....pdf.

Planning Commission. (1981). *Sixth five year plan*. Planning Commission, Government of India. Retrieved from https://niti.gov.in/planningcommission.gov.in/docs/plans/planrel/fiveyr/index7.html.

Planning Commission. (n.d.a). *First five year plan*. Planning Commission, GoI. Retrieved from https://niti.gov.in/planningcommission.gov.in/docs/plans/planrel/fiveyr/index7.html.

Planning Commission. (n.d.b). *Second five year plan*. Planning Commission, GoI. Retrieved from https://niti.gov.in/planningcommission.gov.in/docs/plans/planrel/fiveyr/index7.html.

Planning Commission. (n.d.c). *Third five year plan*. Planning Commission, GoI. Retrieved from https://niti.gov.in/planningcommission.gov.in/docs/plans/planrel/fiveyr/index7.html.

Planning Commission. (n.d.d). *Fourth five year plan*. Planning Commission, GoI. Retrieved from https://niti.gov.in/planningcommission.gov.in/docs/plans/planrel/fiveyr/index7.html.

Planning Commission. (n.d.e). *Fifth five year plan*. Planning Commission, GoI. Retrieved from https://niti.gov.in/planningcommission.gov.in/docs/plans/planrel/fiveyr/index7.html.

Planning Commission. (n.d.f). Housing, urban development and water supply. *Sixth five year plan*. Planning Commission, Government of India. Retrieved from https://niti.gov.in/planningcommission.gov.in/docs/plans/planrel/fiveyr/6th/6planch23.html.

Planning Commission. (n.d.g). *Seventh five year plan* (Vol. 2). Planning Commission, GoI. Retrieved from https://niti.gov.in/planningcommission.gov.in/docs/plans/planrel/fiveyr/index7.html.

Planning Commission. (n.d.h). *Eighth five year plan* (Vol. 2). Planning Commission, GoI. Retrieved from https://niti.gov.in/planningcommission.gov.in/docs/plans/planrel/fiveyr/index7.html.

Planning Commission. (n.d.i). *Ninth five year plan* (Vol. 2). Planning Commission, GoI. Retrieved from https://niti.gov.in/planningcommission.gov.in/docs/plans/planrel/fiveyr/index7.html.

Planning Commission. (n.d.j). *Sector policies and programmes. Tenth five year plan* (Vol. 2). Planning Commission, GoI. Retrieved from https://www.niti.gov.in/planningcommission.gov.in/docs/plans/planrel/fiveyr/10th/volume2/10th_vol2.pdf.

Planning Commission. (n.d.k). *Twelfth five year plan*. Planning Commission, GoI. Retrieved from https://niti.gov.in/planningcommission.gov.in/docs/plans/planrel/fiveyr/12th/pdf/12fyp_vol1.pdf.

Pol, E., & Ville, S. (2009). Social innovation: Buzz word or enduring term? *Journal of Socio-Economics*, *38*(6), 878–885.

Pradhan, G. R. (1938). *Untouchable workers of Bombay city*. Karnatak Publishing House. Retrieved from https://www.readbookpage.com/pdf/untouchable -workers-of-bombay-city.

Prashad, V. (1995). Between economism and emancipation: Untouchables and Indian Nationalism, 1920–1950. *Left History*, 3(1), 5–30. Retrieved from https://www.scribd.com/document/210277733/Between-Economism-and -Emancipation.

Primo, N. (2010). *Communication for influence: Linking advocacy, dissemination and research by building ICTD networks in Central, East and West Africa (CICEWA) project, 2008–2010: An evaluation of influence and advocacy*. Canada's International Development Research Centre (IDRC). Retrieved from https://www.apc.org/sites/default/files/CICEWA_Advocacy_Evaluation_0.pdf.

Quebral, N. (2001). New dimensions, bold decisions. In *Development communication in a borderless world*. Continuing Education Centre, Department of Science Communication, College of Development Communication, University of the Philippines.

Rahman, M. A. (1982). The theory and practice of participatory action research. Paper prepared for Plenary Session on "Contradictions, Conflicts and Strategies of Societal Change", at the Tenth World Congress of Sociology; Rural Employment Policies Branch, Employment and Development Department, ILO, Geneva.

Ramaiah, A. (2011). Growing crimes against Dalits in India despite special laws: Relevance of Ambedkar's demand for 'separate settlement. *Journal of Law and Conflict Resolution*, 3(9), 151–168. https://doi.org/10.5897/JLCR10.033.

Ramani, S. V., SadreGhazi, S., & Gupta, S. (2017). Catalysing innovation for social impact: The role of social enterprises in the Indian Sanitation Sector. *Technological Forecasting and Social Change*, 121, 216–227. Retrieved from http://finishsociety .org/upload-image/Annual-File/1536600800_Social%20Enterprises%20in %20the%20Indian%20sanitation%20sector%20by%20Dr%20Shyama %20Ramani.pdf.

Rashtriya Garima Abhiyan. (2011). *Eradication of inhuman practice of manual scavenging and Jan Sahas*. Retrieved from https://www.indiawaterportal.org/sites /default/files/iwp2/Eradication_Inhuman_Practice_Manual_Scavenging_India _Rashtriya_Garima_Abhiyaan_2011.pdf.

Rashtriya Garima Abhiyan. (2013). *Maila Mukti Yatra – 2012–13*. Dalit Network Netherlands. Retrieved from http://www.dalits.nl/pdf/MailaMuktiYatra2012 -2013.pdf.

Rogers, E. M. (1976, April). Communication and development: The passing of the dominant paradigm. *Communication Research*, 3(2), 213–240. https://doi.org /10.1177/009365027600300207

Rohilla, S. K., & Trivedi, R. C. (2011). *Policy paper on septage management in India*. Centre for Science and Environment (CSE).

Rosenstock, I. M. (1966, December). Why people use health services. 44, 94–124. https://doi.org/10.1111/j.1468-0009.2005.00425.x.

Schrecongost, A., Pedi, D., Rosenboom, J. W., Shrestha, R., & Radu, B. (2020). Citywide inclusive sanitation: A public service approach for reaching the urban sanitation SDGs. *Frontiers in Environmental Science*, 8, 19.

Schumacher, E. F. (1973). *Small is beautiful: Economics as if people mattered*. Blond and Briggs Lt.

Shahid, M. (2015). Manual scavenging: Issues of caste, culture and violence. *Social Change, 45*(2) 242–255. Retrieved from https://www.academia.edu/41439258/Manual_Scavenging_Issues_of_Caste_Culture_and_Violence.

Sharma, M., & Romas, J. A. (2012). *Theoretical foundations of health education and health promotion.* Jones & Bartlett Learning, LLC.

Shelter Associate. (2008). Conference Paper - Improving Urban Poor's Access to Sanitation: Community-Led Sanitation Program, Sangli, India, Community-Led Sangli Toilet Construction Activity, 33rd WEDC International Conference, Accra, Ghana.

Silvestre, B. S., & Neto, R. e. (2014). Capability accumulation, innovation, and technology diffusion: Lessons from a base of the pyramid cluster. *Technovation, 34*(5–6), May–June 2014, Retrieved from https://www.sciencedirect.com/science/article/abs/pii/S0166497213001120.

Smith, V. (2007). *Clean: A history of personal hygiene and purity.* Oxford University Press.

Soares, J. R. (2020). *Innovation and entrepreneurial opportunities in community tourism.* IGI Global. https://doi.org/10.4018/978-1-7998-4855-4

SQUAT Survey. (2014). *Research institute for compassionate economics (r.i.c.e.), USA.* Retrieved from https://jalshakti-ddws.gov.in/sites/default/files/SQUAT_Survey.pdf.

Stiefel, M., & Wolfe, M. (1994). *A voice for the excluded: Popular participation in development: Utopia or necessity?* Zed Books Ltd.

Sub Group on Safai Karmacharies. (2007). *Working group on the "empowerment of scheduled castes (SCs)" for the eleventh five-year plan (2007–2012).* Retrieved from https://doczz.net/doc/7340360/report-of-sub-group-on-safai-karamcharis

Swachh Bharat Mission - Gramin. (2019). *Department of drinking water and sanitation, Ministry of Jal Shakti, Government of India.* Retrieved from http://sbm.gov.in/sbmreport/home.aspx.

Swachh Bharat Mission - Urban. (2019). *Ministry of housing and urban affairs, Government of India.* Retrieved from: http://swachhbharaturban.gov.in.

Tandon, R. & Bandyopadhyay, K. K.(2004). Capacity building for effective democractic local -governance: Experience from India. PRIA. *Participation and Governance,* (20). 10 (31) pp: 7–16

Tandon, R. (2002). *Voluntary action, civil society, and the state.* Mosaic Books.

Tandon, R., & Bandyopadhyay, K. K. (2003). *Capacity building of Southern NGOs.* Lessons from International Forum on Capacity Building, PRIA.

Tandon, R., & Kak, M. (2007). Participation, civil society, democratic governance and citizenship: A journey of ideas and practices. In Tandon, R. & Kak, M. (eds.), *Citizen participation and democratic governance: In our hands.* Concept Publishing Company.

Teltumbde, A. (2010). Modi spews caste venom. *Economic and Political Weekly, 45*(23), 12–13.

Teltumbde, A. (2014). No Swachh Bharat without annihilation of caste. *Economic and Political Weekly, 49*(45), 11–12.

The Wire. (2018). Seven government surveys to count manual scavengers couldn't agree on how many there are. *The Wire.* Retrieved from https://thewire.in/government/seven-govt-surveys-to-count-manual-scavengers-couldnt-agree-on-how-many-there-are.

Urban Management Centre – UMC. (2014). Generic information system improvement plan (ISIP) for small cities: Water supply system. Performance Assessment System (PAS). Retrieved from https://umcasia.org/wp-content/uploads/01_0009.-Generic-Information-System-Improvement-Plan-ISIP_Water-supply-system-2014_UMC.pdf.

UMC. (2020). Training of sanitation workers on use of personal protective equipment – PPEs. Retrieved from https://umcasia.org/what-we-do/training-of-sanitation-workers-on-use-of-ppes-2.

UMC, & WaterAid India. (2020). *Health, safety and social security challenges of sanitation workers during the COVID-19 pandemic in India.* Retrieved from https://washmatters.wateraid.org/sites/g/files/jkxoof256/files/health-safety-and-social-security-challenges-of-sanitation-workers-during-the-covid-19-pandemic-in-india.pdf.

WaterAid India. (2019). The hidden world of sanitation workers in India. WaterAid India. Retrieved from https://www.wateraidindia.in/sites/g/files/jkxoof336/files/the-hidden-world-of-sanitation-workers-in-india.pdf.

Weimer, D. L., & Vining, A. R. (2017). *Policy analysis concepts and practice.* Routledge. Retrieved from https://www.routledge.com/Policy-Analysis-Concepts-and-Practice/Weimer-Vining/p/book/9781138216518.

WHO, & UNICEF. (2013). *Progress on sanitation and drinking water – 2013 update.* Retrieved from https://www.unwater.org/publications/whounicef-joint-monitoring-programme-water-supply-sanitation-jmp-2013-update.

Wilkins, K. G. (2007). Development communication. *Peace Review*, 8(1), 97–103. https://doi.org/10.1080/10402659608425936.

Wilkins, K. G., & Mody, B. (2001, November). Reshaping development communication: Developing communication and communicating development. *Communication Theory*, 11(4), 385–396. https://doi.org/10.1111/j.1468-2885.2002.tb00249.x.

World Bank. (2011). World bank open data. Population, total. Retrieved from https://data.worldbank.org/indicator/SP.POP.TOTL?end=2011&start=1960.

World Bank. (2013a). World bank open data. GDP per capita (US$). Retrieved from https://data.worldbank.org/indicator/NY.GDP.PCAP.CD.

World Bank. (2013b). World bank open data. Mortality rate, infant (per 1000 live births). Retrieved from https://data.worldbank.org/indicator/SP.DYN.IMRT.IN.

World Health Organization (WHO). (2008). *Cancer control: Knowledge into action.* WHO. Retrieved from https://www.ncbi.nlm.nih.gov/books/NBK195422.

Young, E., & Quinn, L. (2012). *Making research evidence matter.* Open Society Foundation. Retrieved from https://advocacyguide.icpolicyadvocacy.org/21-defining-policy-advocacy.

Zapf, W. (1991). The role of innovations in modernization theory. *International Review of Sociology*, 2(3), 83–94.

# Index

Page numbers in *italics* indicate figures and **bold** indicate tables in the text.

For Product Safety Concerns and Information please contact our EU
representative  GPSR@taylorandfrancis.com
Taylor & Francis Verlag GmbH, Kaufingerstraße 24, 80331 München, Germany

www.ingramcontent.com/pod-product-compliance
Lightning Source LLC
Chambersburg PA
CBHW060307220326
41598CB00027B/4256